THE
EVERYDAY
DIABETIC
COOKBOOK

STELLA BOWLING

GRUB STREET · LONDON

Published by Grub Street, 4 Rainham Close
London SW11 6SS

Original edition published 1995
Copyright this edition © Grub Street 2001
Text copyright © Diabetes UK 2001

Reprinted 1997, 1998 (twice), 1999, 2000 (twice), 2001 (three times)
2002, 2003, 2004 (twice), 2005, 2006, 2007, 2008, 2009, 2010, 2011,
2012, 2013

British Library Cataloguing in Publication Data
Bowling, Stella
  Everyday Diabetic Cookbook
  I. Title
  641.56314

ISBN 978 1 898697 25 1

Edited by Fiona Eves
Illustrations by Madeleine David
Photography by Tim Imrie
Food preparation and styling by Anne Dolamore
Typesetting by Pearl Graphics, Hemel Hempstead
Printed and bound in Great Britain by
Berforts Information Press Ltd.

Grub Street only uses FSC (Forest Stewardship Council) paper for
its books

Contents

ACKNOWLEDGEMENTS

I would like to thank my colleagues at Diabetes UK in the Care Development Team for making the book possible.

The text explaining about diabetes is taken from the Diabetes UK leaflet 'Understanding diabetes – your key to better health', one of a range of comprehensive information booklets produced by Diabetes UK on every aspect of diabetes.

The most thanks go to my husband Karl for his encouragement and patience, as well as his constructive comments. Thanks also to my nieces Katie and Amy Hancock and my cousin Emma Thomas for their tasting skills and comments on the children's recipes. And last but not least, thanks to my baby daughter Jade for sleeping enough in her early weeks to allow me to test the recipes!

Preface

Food and eating are part of life's great pleasures. Having diabetes doesn't need to change that. Today, people with diabetes are advised to eat a wide variety of healthy foods and nothing is completely taboo. It doesn't mean you have to give up all of your favourite foods completely nor not try interesting meals and new recipes. What is more important is eating a balanced diet with a wide variety of foods and having increased awareness of which foods promote good health, and which foods should be eaten only in moderation.

As you will see from this book, the diet for people with diabetes is the same as the diet recommended for everyone – low in fat, sugar and salt with plenty of fruit and vegetables.

The Everyday Diabetic Cookbook shows you how easy and enjoyable healthy eating can be and provides a wide range of recipes to help you put healthy eating for diabetes into practice. But, before you start cooking, we will look at diabetes in more detail.

DIABETES UK
(the new name for the British Diabetic Association)

There are 1.4 million people diagnosed with diabetes in the UK. It is estimated there are as many as a million who do not know they have the condition. Although it cannot be prevented or cured, medication and an appropriate diet can control it.

Diabetes UK has been advising and helping people with diabetes for over 65 years. Founded by the author HG Wells and Dr RD Lawrence in 1934, Diabetes UK was the first self-help group for people with diabetes in the UK. Its aims then were the same as they are today: to support and inform people with diabetes and to support diabetes research.

Diabetes UK also produces a range of award winning publications about all aspects of diabetes care – many of them free. For a catalogue of our publications freephone 0800 585088.

Diabetes UK is the charity for people with diabetes and has a membership of over 190,000 with more than 400 voluntary groups throughout the country. Among other benefits, members of Diabetes UK receive *Balance*, Diabetes UK's lively magazine, free every two months and it is available on tape for the visually impaired.

The Government recognises Diabetes UK as the official voice of diabetes in the UK and MPs have formed an All-Party Parliamentary Group for diabetes.

Diabetes UK is the major funder of research dedicated to diabetes in the UK, spending almost £4.5m on research annually, received through subscriptions and donations.

If you would like to find out more about Diabetes UK or would like to become a member, please contact Diabetes UK Customer Services on 020 7462 2791. To discuss diabetes-related problems, please contact Diabetes UK Careline on 020 7636 6112 (operates an interpretation service) or by textphone: 020 7462 2757, fax: 020 7637 3644, email: careline@diabetes.org.uk

Or write to us at:
10 Queen Anne Street
London
W1G 9LH

DIABETES AND A HEALTHY LIFESTYLE

WHAT IS DIABETES?

Diabetes or, to give it its full name, diabetes mellitus, is a common condition in which the amount of glucose (sugar) in the blood is too high because the body is unable to use it properly. This is because the body's method of converting glucose into energy is not working as it should. Normally the amount of glucose in our blood is carefully controlled by a hormone called insulin. Insulin is made by a gland called the pancreas which lies just behind the stomach. It helps the glucose to enter the cells where it is used as fuel by the body. Diabetes develops when there is a shortage of insulin or when the body's insulin doesn't work properly.

We obtain glucose from the food that we eat, either from sweet foods or from the digestion of starchy foods such as bread or potatoes. Glucose can also be made by the liver. After a meal, the blood glucose level rises and insulin is released into the blood. When the blood glucose level falls (for example, during exercise), the level of insulin falls. Insulin, therefore, plays a vital role in regulating the level of glucose in the blood and, in particular, in stopping that blood glucose level from rising too high.

There are two main types of diabetes:

Type 1 (insulin dependent) diabetes

Type 2 diabetes (non insulin dependent) diabetes

Type 1 diabetes

Type 1 diabetes develops when there is a severe lack of insulin in the body because most or all of the cells (in the pancreas) which produce it have been destroyed. This type of diabetes usually appears in people under the age of 40, often in childhood. It is treated by insulin injections and diet.

Type 2 diabetes

Type 2 diabetes develops when the body can still produce some insulin, though not enough for its needs, or when the insulin that the body does produce is not working properly (known as insulin resistance). This type of diabetes usually appears in people over the age of 40, though it often appears before the age of 40 in South Asian and African-Caribbean people. It is treated by diet and exercise alone, by diet and tablets or sometimes by diet and insulin injections.

What are the symptoms of diabetes?
The main symptoms of diabetes are:

– Increased thirst

– Going to the loo all the time – especially during the night

– Extreme tiredness

– Weight loss

– Itching genitals or regular episodes of thrush

– Blurred vision

Type 2 diabetes develops slowly and the symptoms are usually less severe. People sometimes put the symptoms down to 'getting older' or 'overwork'. Other people may not notice any symptoms at all but their diabetes is picked up in a routine medical check-up.

Type 1 diabetes develops much more quickly, usually over a few weeks. Both types of diabetes are serious but the symptoms are quickly relieved once the diabetes is treated. When the diabetes is well controlled, there is no reason why people with diabetes can't lead a healthy and active life. Delayed treatment, however, can lead to complications such as blindness, kidney failure, and heart disease.

WHO GETS DIABETES AND WHAT CAUSES IT?
Diabetes is a common health condition. In the UK, about 1.4 million people in the UK are known to have diabetes and another estimated one million people don't know they have it. More than three-quarters of people with diabetes have Type 2 diabetes. Type 1 diabetes is most often diagnosed in children and young people under 15, although it can occur at any age.

Type 1 diabetes
As mentioned earlier, Type 1 diabetes develops when the insulin producing cells in the pancreas have been destroyed. Nobody knows for sure why these cells have been damaged. But the most likely cause is an abnormal reaction of the body against the cells. This may be triggered by a viral or other infection. It generally affects younger people. Both sexes are equally affected.

Type 2 diabetes
Type 2 diabetes used to be called 'maturity onset' diabetes because it usually appears in middle-aged or elderly people, although it is increasingly common in younger people. The main cause is that the body no longer responds normally to its own insulin. Some people wrongly describe this as 'mild' diabetes. But all diabetes should be taken seriously and treated properly.

The people most at risk of developing Type 2 diabetes are those with a family history of diabetes, people aged between 40 and 75, South Asian or African-Caribbean people, people who are very overweight and women who have had 'gestational diabetes' or have given birth to a large baby.

There are some other causes of diabetes but they are all very rare. They include certain diseases of the pancreas. Sometimes, an accident or an illness may reveal diabetes if it is already there, but they do not cause it. Diabetes is not caused by eating sweets or the wrong kind of food. Stress does not cause diabetes although it may make the symptoms worse if it is already there. You cannot catch diabetes from somebody, nor can you give it to them.

HOW IS DIABETES TREATED?

Although diabetes cannot yet be 'cured', it can be treated very successfully. Before discussing the different kinds of treatment, it is important to know something about blood glucose levels.

When sugary and starchy foods have been digested, they turn into glucose. As we have seen, when somebody has diabetes, the glucose in their body is not turned into energy because there is not enough insulin (or because the insulin that the body is producing is not being used properly). So the liver makes more glucose than usual. However, this also cannot be turned into energy. The body then breaks down its stores of fat and protein to try and release more glucose but this, too, cannot be turned into energy. This is why people with untreated diabetes often feel tired and lose weight. The unused glucose spills over into the urine – which is why people with untreated diabetes need to pass urine more often. Type 1 diabetes is treated by injections of insulin and a healthy diet. Type 2 diabetes is treated by a healthy diet and exercise or often by a combination of a healthy diet and tablets. Sometimes people with Type 2 diabetes also take insulin injections, although they are still producing some insulin themselves.

Type 1 diabetes

People with Type 1 diabetes need to take injections of insulin for the rest of their lives and they need to eat a healthy diet that contains the right balance of foods. Insulin cannot be swallowed like a medicine because it is destroyed by the digestive juices in the stomach. A flexible regimen with up to four injections each day may be used. If you or someone close to you needs to take insulin injections, your doctor or diabetes specialist nurse will talk to you, show you how to do them and give you all the support and help you need. They will also show you how you can do a simple blood or urine test at home to measure your blood glucose levels so that you can adjust your insulin and diet according to your daily routine. They will advise what to do if your glucose level is too low. If you have this type of diabetes, injections of insulin are necessary to keep you alive and you need to take them every day.

Type 2 diabetes

People with Type 2 diabetes need to eat a healthy diet that contains the right balance of foods. If your doctor or diabetes specialist nurse finds that this alone is not enough to keep your blood glucose levels normal, you may be given tablets to take. There are several types of diabetes tablets. Some help your pancreas to produce more insulin while others help your body to make better use of the insulin that your pancreas is producing. Sometimes a combination of tablets is used. Your doctor or diabetes specialist nurse will tell you all about the tablets, when to take them, and how to monitor your blood or urine glucose levels.

HEALTHY EATING

The diet recommended for people with diabetes is not a special diet; it is a healthy balanced diet that is recommended for everybody – low in fat, sugar and salt, with plenty of fruit and vegetables. What you eat directly affects your blood glucose levels. It can also influence the amount of fat (such as cholesterol) in your blood. So it is important to eat the right kind of foods to stay healthy.

Six steps to eating a healthy diet

1. Eat regular meals based on starchy foods such as bread, pasta, chapatis, potatoes, rice and cereals. This will help you control your blood glucose levels. Choose high fibre varieties of these foods like wholemeal bread and wholewheat cereals more often.

2. Try to cut down on the fat you eat, particularly saturated animal fats, as this type of fat is linked to heart disease. Eating less fat and fatty foods will also help you lose weight. Choose low fat dairy foods like skimmed milk and low fat yogurt. Grill, steam or oven bake rather than frying food.

3. Eat more fruit and vegetables – aim for at least five portions a day to provide you with vitamins and fibre as well as to help balance your overall diet.

4. Cut down on sugar and sugary foods. This does not mean you need to try to eat a sugar-free diet. Use diet, low-sugar or sugar-free squashes and fizzy drinks as sugary drinks cause blood glucose levels to rise quickly.

5. Use less salt. Try flavouring foods with herbs and spices rather than adding salt.

6. Drink alcohol in moderation only – that's two units of alcohol a day for a woman and three units a day for a man. Remember never drink on an empty stomach as alcohol can increase the likelihood of hypoglycaemia (low blood glucose levels). And never drink and drive.

As you can see from the recommendations, there is no need for 'special' or 'diabetic' foods because you have diabetes. Diabetic products are not recommended as there is no evidence that these foods offer any special advantage to people with diabetes. They are not felt to be necessary as part of a healthy-eating plan and may also prove expensive.

Your dietitian or diabetes healthcare team will be able to discuss with you the right amount of food for you. They may also advise you on changing the way you cook some foods or on altering some of the ingredients in your recipes (for example by using a different fat or oil), or that you may need to eat less of certain foods. However, the basic foods themselves will mostly be those that you have always eaten.

PUTTING HEALTHY EATING INTO PRACTICE

You may be wondering how all this advice relates to you and your day-to-day eating plan. Dietary management of diabetes depends on eating regularly, basing meals on starchy carbohydrate foods and including more fruit, vegetables and pulses in your everyday diet.

No one is expected to make drastic changes overnight! This would be very disheartening. Instead make the changes gradually by making one or two amendments a week. For example, if you need to cut down on fat in your diet you could substitute a low-fat spread or a reduced-fat monounsaturated spread in place of margarine or butter one week, and then change from using a full-fat milk to skimmed or semi-skimmed milk in the following weeks. You will soon find that you are eating balanced meals every day, which are enjoyable too.

Variety is also an important factor as no single food contains all the nutrients your body needs in the amounts required, but some foods (such as very fatty or sugary foods) should not be eaten too often, or in large quantities if you want to ensure a balanced diet. So you have to eat a mixture of foods to get the right amount of nutrients.

This is made easier if you choose foods from each of the five food groups each day – starchy foods; dairy products; meat, poultry, fish and alternatives; vegetables and fruit and fatty and sugary foods. Follow the chart below, which shows the proportions of types of food to fill your plate for a healthy balanced diet.

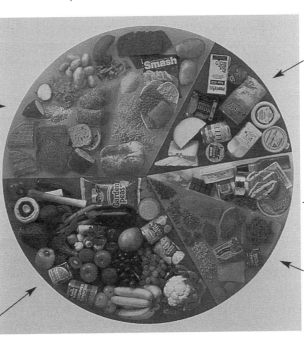

Bread, cereals, rice, pasta and potatoes: base all meals and snacks on starchy foods. Choose wholemeal and whole-grain varieties whenever possible.

Milk and dairy foods: choose lower fat versions of dairy foods for adults.

Fatty and sugary foods: cut down on sugary and fatty foods.

Fruit and vegetables: choose a wide variety of foods from this group.

Meat, fish and alternatives: eat a variety of different foods from this group and choose lower fat alternatives whenever possible.

BASE YOUR MEALS ON STARCHY CARBOHYDRATE FOODS

As we have seen, starchy carbohydrate foods should form the basis of your meals with fruit and vegetables making up one third to half of your plate. A simple way of ensuring this is to let the starchy component of your meal fill about half your plate and meat, fish or cheese (ie the protein foods), the smaller part.

Many people believe that people with diabetes have to cut right down on starchy carbohydrate foods such as bread, potatoes, pasta, rice and chapatis, but this is not true. Some people are advised to eat snacks between meals to spread the starchy carbohydrate intake more evenly throughout the day.

Eating plenty of these starchy carbohydrate foods as part of a generally healthy and varied diet helps to control your blood glucose.

Include more low glycaemic index (GI) foods

Although you may not have heard of the term 'GI' before, you may already have been encouraged to include low GI foods such as beans and pulses in your diet. Low GI foods can help to improve blood glucose control as they cause a slow steady rise in blood glucose levels and also curb your appetite by making you feel fuller for longer.

It was previously thought that if you ate the same amount of carbohydrate, whatever it was, it would have the same effect on your blood glucose levels. It is now known that different carbohydrate-containing foods have different effects on blood glucose levels. For example, 30 g of carbohydrate as bread do not have exactly the same effect as 30 g of carbohydrate as fruit or 30 g of carbohydrate as pasta.

Foods are given a GI number according to their effect on blood glucose levels. Glucose or white bread (50 g) is used as the standard reference (GI 100), and other foods are measured against this by comparing the effect of a 50 g portion of the test food on blood glucose levels.

The GI of a food is affected by many things such as cooking, texture, drink as well as the other foods it is being eaten with. One food is rarely eaten alone, for example oats are eaten with milk, baked beans are usually eaten on toast and so on. This makes it not particularly useful to look at specific values in isolation and since the GI will change with the addition of different foods, it can be difficult and extremely complex to estimate the overall impact of a meal. The principle is that by eating lower GI foods with higher ones, this will lower the overall GI effect of a meal, eg meringue following a pasta meal is better than meringue on its own.

Diabetes UK's view is that the simplest approach in the application of the GI is to combine meals with fruit, vegetables and high fibre starchy foods like cereals and pulses in order to achieve a better blood glucose control. In effect this is what our dietary guidelines suggest already, to base all meals on starchy carbohydrate foods, including high fibre varieties. However this does not mean that foods with a medium or high GI need to be excluded.

GI ratings

Low: fruit, beans, lentils, pasta (all types made from durum wheat), barley, basmati rice, porridge, custard.

Medium: honey, jam, Shredded Wheat, Weetabix, ice-cream, new potatoes.

High: glucose, white and wholemeal bread, brown rice, cornflakes, baked potatoes, mashed potato.

Low GI meal plan

Including a low GI food with each meal will lower the overall GI content of the meal.

Breakfast: use an oat-based breakfast cereal and eat some fruit. Muesli and All Bran are also good choices.

Snacks: yogurt, fruit, popcorn, rye bread, fruit loaf. Be careful of some foods that have a lower GI as they may be high in fat (chocolate and nuts) or sugar (fruit yogurt).

Lunch: add baked beans to a jacket potato or try a lentil-based soup. Add variety with different breads, such as pitta, pumpernickel and breads with a substantial amount of mixed grain.

Evening meal: basmati rice, sweet potato, buckwheat, bulgar wheat, pearl barley and noodles are good accompaniments to meals. Eat more pasta-based meals and include more beans and pulses.

Fibre

Fibre is simply the part of food that you don't digest and used to be referred to as roughage. Foods high in fibre usually contain a mixture of insoluble and soluble fibre.

Insoluble fibre helps you to maintain a healthy digestive system and reduces the risks of developing bowel disorders such as diverticulitis and haemorrhoids and helps to prevent constipation. Wholemeal and granary breads, wholewheat breakfast cereals and wholewheat pasta are particularly good sources of insoluble fibre.

Soluble fibre helps to control blood glucose levels by slowing down the rate at which carbohydrates in food get into the blood. It also appears to lower the amount of cholesterol in the blood. Fruit, vegetables, pulses and oats are particularly good sources of soluble fibre.

Beans are also a very good source of soluble fibre (also low-fat source of protein) and there is now a wide selection of tinned beans (such as kidney beans, chickpeas, flageolet beans) available which are easy to prepare and unlike dried beans, do not require soaking overnight.

If you use dried beans, make sure they are cooked properly, following the packet instructions (some are toxic unless they are boiled for at least 10 minutes) and bear in mind that most require soaking for a few hours or, the simplest way, overnight.

Fibre is found in a wide range of foods, but there is no fibre in animal products such as meat, cheese or eggs.

High-fibre starchy foods can also help to control your weight because they are filling without providing too many calories and also take longer to digest. Eating a high-fibre diet does not mean eating wholemeal foods all the time. Combine high and low fibre foods in a meal, eg white rice with a vegetable and lentil curry. For breakfast, fresh or dried fruit can be added to increase the fibre content of lower fibre cereals.

Adding bran to foods to increase your fibre intake is not recommended as bran does not provide the nutrients which are found in foods naturally high in fibre.

Another important aspect to bear in mind when increasing the amount of fibre in your diet is that you will need to drink more fluid. Try to drink at least six to eight cups of water each day. It is also wise to increase the amount of fibre in your diet gradually as it may upset your digestive system if you suddenly consume a lot more fibre than your body is used to.

Hints to increase fibre in your diet

- Choose wholemeal or granary breads rather than white bread, wholemeal pittas or chapatis or try a high-fibre white bread.

- Eat plenty of fruit, vegetables (at least five servings per day) and pulses such as peas, beans and lentils.

- Leave skins on potatoes.

- Try using more peas, beans and lentils in recipes. In many dishes you can replace some or all of the meat with beans. Try adding lentils to soups, casseroles, etc.

- Try using wholemeal flour in recipes instead of white flour, or try using half wholemeal and half white flour. Using 100 per cent wholemeal flour is unsuitable in some cake recipes where it will give a heavy result.

- Choose fruit-based puddings.

- Add dried or fresh fruit to breakfast cereals.

REDUCE YOUR FAT INTAKE

A small amount of fat in the diet is essential for health and makes food more pleasant to eat. However, most of us eat far more fat than is needed. People with diabetes have a greater risk of developing coronary heart disease and eating less fat is a major factor in reducing this risk. High-fat foods are high in calories so cutting down on them can also help to control your weight.

Semi-skimmed (half-fat) milk tastes like full-fat milk but has had the cream poured off. Skimmed milk has a 'thinner' or more watery taste and may take longer to get used to. Both semi-skimmed and skimmed milks have just as much calcium and protein as whole milk, but have much less fat and calories.

Also available are reduced-fat cheeses and reduced-fat margarines or low-fat spreads. If you already use a polyunsaturated margarine such as 'Flora' this is fine; you may also like to try a monounsaturated spread which is reduced in fat.

Types of fat

There are two main types of fat in foods, saturated and unsaturated. Foods that are high in saturated fats tend to be animal products such as butter, lard, dripping, fatty meat and full-fat dairy products such as cheese and milk. Saturated fats tend to raise the cholesterol in blood, which increases the risk of developing coronary heart disease.

Unsaturated fats include two types – monounsaturated fats and polyunsaturated fats. These fats lower the cholesterol in blood and therefore may help to protect against heart disease. Choose monounsaturated fats in preference to polyunsaturated fats.

Sources of monounsaturated spreads include olive, rapeseed or peanut (groundnut) oil or the reduced-fat monounsaturated spreads and are a better choice than vegetable oils. Examples of reduced-fat monounsaturated spreads include Olivio, Olive Gold and St Ivel Mono.

Polyunsaturated fats are found in oily fish such as herring, mackerel, tuna, pilchards, sardines and trout; corn oil, sunflower, safflower and soya oil and soft margarines or spreads labelled 'high in polyunsaturates'.

Hints to reduce fat

Eat a variety of different protein foods but choose lower fat alternatives whenever possible.

– Choose a spread that is labelled 'high in monounsaturates', in place of butter or hard margarine.

– If you are overweight use a reduced-fat spread, but don't be tempted to put more on because it's lower in fat!

– If you do want to carry on using butter, spread it more thinly.

– Try not using any spread sometimes, for example when serving beans on toast or try having bread the continental way – very fresh with no butter or margarine.

– For adults, use semi-skimmed or skimmed milk, instead of whole (full-fat) milk, for cooking and for drinks and cereals. Both semi-skimmed and skimmed milk have as much calcium and protein as whole milk, but have much less fat and calories.

– Try using low-fat yogurt or very-low-fat fromage frais instead of cream for some dishes. If you do use cream, use less or choose a reduced-fat version, eg half-fat crème fraîche.

– Cut down on cheese, or replace full-fat hard cheese with reduced-fat or low-fat versions. Try cottage cheese or skimmed milk soft cheese in place of full-fat cream cheese.

– Eat cakes, biscuits and pastries in moderation as they are generally high in fat. Some biscuits are available in a lower-fat or 'light' version, but if you only have one or two biscuits as a snack, the fat saving will not be that significant.

– Eat fish more often. Oily fish such as herring, mackerel and sardines are particularly good choices as they contain a beneficial type of fat, Omega 3, which helps protect against heart attack. Oily fish should be eaten at least once a week.

– Buy the leanest cuts of meat you can afford and trim off all the visible fat before cooking. Some supermarkets sell meat that is already trimmed of fat and extra lean minced beef is now widely available.

– Use less meat in recipes and replace or mix it with vegetables, or pulses such as beans or lentils.

– Lentils and beans are an excellent addition to healthy eating, as they are low in fat and a good source of protein and soluble fibre.

– Chicken and turkey are low in fat as long as you remove the skin before eating. Most of the fat is found just under the skin and is easily removed with it.

– Meat products such as sausage rolls, meat pies, beefburgers and sausages are high in fat. Try to cut down on these.

– Cut down on chips or use reduced-fat oven chips instead.

Cooking with less fat
Changing the way you cook can help cut down on added and unnecessary fat in your diet.

– Measure oil with a tablespoon rather than pouring straight from the container, then gradually reduce the amount you use.

– Try to add as little fat as possible when cooking spices for meals such as curries or sautéing vegetables such as onions. You can usually halve the amount called for in most recipes. (The amounts have been reduced in this book.)

– Try stir-frying using a steep-sided, round-bottomed pan like a wok. This allows you to fry your food using only a small amount of oil.

– Invest in a non-stick pan and then you may not need to use any fat or oil at all. For example, when cooking mince, you can 'dry' fry the mince and pour off any excess fat during cooking.

– Try microwaving, steaming, poaching, boiling or grilling instead of roasting and frying.

– Casseroling and stewing are good ways to cook cheaper cuts of meat. Make sure you cut off all visible fat before cooking and drain off fat during cooking. There is no need to fry meat before casseroling, but it may take a little longer to cook.

– Make use of herbs and spices, onions, garlic, or lemon juice instead of butter to flavour foods, particularly vegetables.

– Grill, microwave, steam or bake fish, fishfingers and fishcakes rather than frying or deep-frying.

– Grill beefburgers and sausages rather than frying them.

– Use a rack when roasting meat so that the fat drains off into the roasting pan.

Watch out for hidden fats

You may think of margarine and butter when trying to cut down on fat in your healthy eating plan. However, there are many foods such as meat pies, cakes and biscuits that contain large amounts of fat. This is often referred to as 'hidden' fat. Some of these foods are listed below and you may be surprised at the amount of fat they contain.

Hidden fats

Food	Fat content per average serving
One steak and kidney pie	42 g
A slice of quiche lorraine	39 g
One pork pie	38 g
A serving of macaroni cheese	32 g
A serving of chicken curry	31 g
One medium avocado pear	28 g
One cheese and tomato pizza	27 g
One quarter pounder with cheese	26 g
One fresh cream éclair	21 g
One ring doughnut	16 g
A slice of apple pie	16 g
One rum baba	16 g
A serving of chicken nuggets	14 g
A slice of fresh cream gateau	14 g
One croissant	10 g
Potato crisps (one packet)	9 g
Lower fat crisps (one packet)	7 g

Cholesterol

Cholesterol is made by our bodies and forms part of our cells and tissues. However, too much cholesterol in the blood can lead to a build up of fatty deposits in the arteries, causing heart disease.

Although some foods are naturally high in what is referred to as 'dietary' cholesterol, cutting down on these is not thought to have any significant effect on blood cholesterol levels. Having said that, if you cut down on the total amount of fat, particularly animal fat, you will automatically cut down on cholesterol. It is the total fat intake and types of fat we eat that are important. It is best to cut down on foods that are high in saturated fats, or replace them with monounsaturated or polyunsaturated fats and oils as saturated fat raises blood cholesterol levels.

EAT MORE FRUIT AND VEGETABLES

Choose a wide variety of foods from this group. The UK diet tends to be particularly low in fruits and vegetables and the World Health Organisation (WHO) and Diabetes UK both recommend a target of five portions of fruit and vegetables a day. Fruit and vegetables are important to include in your diet as they contain valuable vitamins, minerals and, as discussed on pages 7-8, fibre.

Many people are concerned about eating fruit because of the natural sugar it contains, for example you may have been told not to eat too many grapes. This is because grapes are very sweet and you could easily eat a whole bunch, as they are 'more-ish'. All fruit whether fresh, frozen, dried or tinned in juice is fine. Spread your intake between meals and snacks over the whole day.

Fruit and vegetables may actually reduce risk of coronary heart disease and as we have one of the highest rates of coronary heart disease, this is another good reason to try and eat more of these. Vitamin C is one of the antioxidant vitamins; others are vitamin A and E. Antioxidants are believed to have a neutralising effect on the cell-damaging free-radical compounds in the body and therefore help to keep us healthy. Free radicals are created during the everyday chemical reactions within the body.

It is particularly important to try to have some foods rich in vitamin C every day as it is a water-soluble vitamin and cannot be stored in the body. This nutrient is also used up faster during times of stress, which may explain why colds and infections seem to strike when we are feeling run down or not eating properly. Good natural sources of vitamin C are citrus fruits such as oranges, lemons and grapefruits as well as blackcurrants, rosehips, green peppers, parsley, potatoes and most fresh fruit and vegetables.

Vitamin A, another antioxidant nutrient is fat soluble and can be stored in the body until needed, but it is still a good idea to keep reserves topped up. Good sources are liver and oily fish. Vitamin A can also be made in the body from beta carotene which is plentiful in yellow or orange coloured fruits and vegetables such as carrots, apricots, oranges and dark green vegetables such as spinach, spring greens and broccoli.

Vitamin E is found in tomatoes, sweet potatoes, chickpeas, wholegrain breads and cereals and certain oils such as corn oil.

There are many other beneficial substances in fruit and vegetables which is why you should eat plenty of them rather than taking vitamin pills.

CUT DOWN ON SUGAR AND SUGARY FOODS

Lots of foods contain sugar, either natural or added but it's the overall food choices you make that determine whether you have a balanced diet.

Many people believe that they will have to cut out sugar completely when they are diagnosed with diabetes, but this is not necessary. It is best to avoid concentrated forms of sugar such as sugary soft drinks and sweets. These can make your blood glucose level rise quickly, which is undesirable, except when treating hypoglycaemia (low blood glucose level), or a 'hypo'. Sugar taken as part of a meal is not detrimental to diabetes control, as it is eaten mixed in with other foods so will be absorbed more slowly into the body.

With regards to homemade cakes and biscuits, Diabetes UK recommends the use of ordinary sugar where nothing else adequately replaces the bulk and creaming qualities of sugar. In cake recipes, the amount of sugar required can sometimes be reduced by up to half. There is advice on pages 17-18 on how to adapt your own favourite recipes. Or you can try the tested reduced-sugar recipes in this book.

Many sugary foods are also high in fat and calories, for example chocolate and cream cakes. Cakes, biscuits, chocolates and sweets are not a large part of a balanced diet so it is a good idea to have these only occasionally, especially if you are trying to lose weight.

Tooth decay is another reason to limit these foods. Eating sugar is the main cause of tooth decay, especially when sugary foods and drinks are eaten frequently through the day.

Hints to eat less sugar

– Drink tea and coffee without sugar. If you are used to having a lot of sugar in drinks, you may find it easier to cut down a little at a time. If you can't get used to drinks without sweetness, try using an intense (artificial) sweetener.

– When buying soft drinks, choose low-calorie or diet drinks, rather than the 'regular' versions which raise the blood glucose levels quickly.

– Choosing ordinary jam won't be detrimental to your overall blood glucose control as the amount you use is only small so won't affect the overall control. Choose reduced sugar if you prefer.

– Low-sugar or sugar-free desserts such as tinned fruit in juice rather than syrup, sugar-free dessert whips such as Angel Delight or sugar-free jelly can help reduce the overall sugar content of your diet.

Intense (artificial) sweeteners
Intense or artificial sweeteners provide an intense level of sweetness when only a minute quantity is used. As a result, they are often referred to as 'intense' sweeteners. Intense sweeteners are available in different forms – tablets, granulated or liquid. They also have different tastes and sweetening capacity, so it is advisable to shop around to find a brand that suits your particular needs. These are virtually calorie-free and can be used at home in hot and cold drinks, to sprinkle onto cereals and stewed fruit. They are also found in many manufactured products such as sugar-free desserts, diet yogurts, sugar-free gum, diet fizzy drinks and low-calorie squash.

Different types of intense sweeteners
Tablet sweeteners are best used for sweetening hot or cold drinks. Each tablet has the sweetening strength of one teaspoon of sugar. So if you usually have two teaspoons of sugar in a cup of tea, you would need to use around two tablets to give the same sweetness. Everyone's perception of sweetness is different. In many cases – sweeten to taste.

Granulated sweeteners contain bulking agents that allow them to be used just like ordinary sugar. For example, one teaspoon of sugar would be replaced by one teaspoon of granulated sweetener.

Liquid sweeteners are very intense and eight to ten drops are equivalent to a teaspoon of sugar.

Are all sweeteners suitable for baking?

Diabetes UK does not recommend the use of intense sweeteners in baking. There is no real substitute for ordinary sugar when it comes to baking as intense sweeteners do not provide the bulk required so the end result can be flat and heavy. They also tend to turn bitter on heating.

Cakes and biscuits form only a small part of a balanced diet as they are generally high in fat and calories. Therefore ordinary sugar can be used without upsetting long-term blood glucose control.

USE LESS SALT

Cutting down on salt can improve high blood pressure in some people and is also associated with reducing the risk of heart disease and stroke. Well-controlled blood pressure (and well-controlled blood glucose levels) has been shown to help reduce the risk of long-term complications of diabetes.

Hints to reduce salt intake

–   Cut down on salty food such as crisps, salty snack foods and smoked meats and fish.

–   Use fewer tinned, packaged and processed foods such as packet soups which are often high in salt content.

–   Look for reduced salt foods where possible.

–   Avoid adding extra salt at the table and use less in cooking. Cut down gradually on the amount used so you can get used to any change in taste. Most of the recipes in this book call for salt to taste and have been tested without any, or using minimum of salt only.

–   Use other flavourings in place of salt such as pepper, garlic, fresh herbs, etc.

DRINK ALCOHOL IN MODERATION ONLY

If you have diabetes there should be no reason why you cannot enjoy a drink, unless of course you have been advised to avoid alcohol as it is high in calories. Alcohol has little or no nutrients and does not therefore contribute to a healthy eating plan. The recommended maximum alcohol intake for people with diabetes is the same as for everyone. This is three units a day for men and two units a day for women. It is also desirable to have two or three days a week without alcohol.

One unit of alcohol = 1/2 pint (275 ml) ordinary strength beer, lager or cider

1 pub measure of sherry, vermouth, aperitif or liqueur

1 standard glass of wine

1 pub measure of spirit, for example gin or vodka

If you are taking certain tablets or insulin for your diabetes, alcohol can contribute to a hypo. Drinking alcohol also makes it harder to recognise a hypo and recover from it. It is therefore important to bear in mind the following:

- Don't drink on an empty stomach or miss a meal so that you can have a drink.
- If you drink beer or lager, choose the ordinary ones. Low-sugar 'diet' beers and lagers tend to be higher in alcohol and so are of no benefit over ordinary ones.
- Low-alcohol beers and lagers may be useful in keeping your alcohol intake down. However, it is best to check the amount of alcohol in each drink even when drinking only low-alcohol drinks.
- Try to use sugar-free or Slimline mixers rather than the ordinary mixers such as tonic water or lemonade.
- If you drink wine or sherry, choose the medium or dry varieties when you can, although the occasional sweet drink would be fine.
- Always wear some form of diabetes identification or carry a Diabetes UK ID card (available from Diabetes UK Customer Services).
- Bear in mind that all types of alcoholic drinks are high in calories.
- If you are overweight, or trying to lose weight, it is best to have only the occasional drink.
- You may be at risk of having a hypo several hours after drinking alcohol. It is important therefore to have something to eat before, with, or shortly after drinking alcohol. If you have had several drinks throughout the evening, it would be best to have a substantial bedtime snack.
- Never drink and drive.

A GUIDE TO SHOPPING

The myth that people with diabetes shouldn't eat any sugar still persists but the truth is that people with diabetes can eat sugar. Although sugar should be limited as part of a healthy diet, good blood glucose control can still be achieved when sugar, and sugar-containing foods are eaten. Dietary management of diabetes depends more on eating regularly, basing meals on starchy carbohydrate foods like pasta and including more fruit, vegetables and pulses in your everyday diet. The main thing to consider is the overall balance of what you're eating – with the emphasis on long-term health and weight control.

Know your labels

When buying ready-made meals and manufactured foods, the nutritional labelling can often help you to make healthier choices. Convenience foods can be useful as a time saving option and needn't always be unhealthy.

Ready-made meals and sauces tend to be high in fat and salt and low in fibre. Choose lower fat or healthy choice options, especially if they are eaten regularly or in larger quantities, as they will affect your overall diet. Vegetarian choices are not necessarily any healthier and can be high in fat. Always serve with extra vegetables or salad, and extra starchy carbohydrate if needed.

Some foods do contain a lot of fat, sugar or calories but if you only eat them occasionally (eg fruit pie) or in small amounts (eg jam) then the fat, sugar and calories won't be significant in your overall diet.

The ingredients list can help you know what is in the food. For example, whether sugar has been added to the food or whether it occurs naturally. But it doesn't tell you how much of an ingredient is used and it may put you off a good choice. For example, sugar is often near the beginning of the ingredients list on products, but this doesn't necessarily mean there's a lot of sugar in it.

Healthy eating logos

These are used in healthy eating ranges produced by supermarkets. Foods may be lower in fat, sugar or salt, or higher in fibre – but not necessarily all of these. These logos can help identify healthier options but you still have to think about how the food fits into your diet.

EATING OUT

Having diabetes should not disrupt your lifestyle. There is no reason why you cannot enjoy the pleasures of dining out or eating away from home. Remember that if you only eat out on special occasions, you should not feel guilty about eating something that you would not normally eat, or if you over indulge a little. If you are watching your weight, it is best to try and avoid the menu choices that are high in fat and calories. But don't worry, there are usually other suitable dishes to choose from.

If you eat out frequently, for example, several times a week, then you will probably need to think more carefully about the foods you choose. Try to avoid very rich or creamy sauces, too many fried foods or sweet desserts. Watch the amount of alcohol you have too.

Here are some hints that you may find helpful when choosing from the menu.

–   Choose main course dishes that are lower in fat and calories. Try to avoid fried dishes and those served with lots of butter or in rich sauces or dressings.

–   Include generous portions of fresh vegetables or salad with your meal.

–   Boiled or jacket potatoes are a healthier choice than chips. If you do choose chips have a small portion and fill up with a bread roll as well.

–   Bear in mind that most desserts at a restaurant are usually high in fat and possibly sugar. This doesn't mean you can have only fresh fruit, but you may have to choose more carefully.

– Cheese and biscuits may seem a virtuous end to a meal, but remember that this choice can be high in fat and calories. Choose only a small selection of cheese and biscuits if you prefer to end your meal this way.

Occasional indulgence in a meal when eating out may cause a temporary rise in your blood glucose level, but will not do any long-term harm. It is the day-to-day control that is important. However, if you are concerned about eating out, it may be helpful to ask your dietician or healthcare team for some guidance. With some experience and some trial and error, you will soon become more confident about what dishes to choose when dining away from home.

ABOUT THE RECIPES

All the recipes in this cookbook have been adapted, where possible, to be lower in fat and in sugar and high in fibre.

Each recipe has been carefully tried and tested using ingredients that are all easily available from supermarkets. As well as good nutrition, taste, variety and enjoyment of food have certainly not been forgotten and are considered as absolutely essential when following a healthy-eating plan.I hope you will agree that there are recipes to suit various occasions and palates with an emphasis on the Mediterranean-style of eating, although some are considered classic favourites that you will recognise.

ADAPTING YOUR OWN RECIPES

The healthy diet for people with diabetes is the healthy diet for everyone – regardless of whether you have diabetes or not. Although people with diabetes do not need special recipes, our recipes have been devised to make them lower in fat, salt and sugar and higher in fibre but still deliciously appetising. Our tips will also help you to modify your own recipes. We have taken care to make the recipes quick and easy to prepare to help you decide what you need to eat to balance your meals. We've provided the nutrition information for each recipe per serving.

The recipes in this book will give you some ideas. With a little practice you will soon find it easy to adapt your own family favourites to be lower in fat and lower in sugar, without compromising on taste. The following hints should help:

– When filling cakes try to use lower fat alternatives to whipped double cream or butter cream. For instance, you can use a mixture of whipped whipping cream and yogurt, or light crème fraîche with fresh fruit.

– Replace some of the white flour in the recipe with wholemeal – up to a half will give good results, but more than this can give a heavy result. For plainer cakes such as Victoria sandwich or Madeira, keep to white flour as this gives the best results.

– Using a low-fat or reduced-fat spread in place of butter or margarine will reduce the fat and calories. However, low-fat spreads are not suitable for all recipes, in which case polyunsaturated margarines or monounsaturated spreads are a useful alternative. Standard margarines have exactly the same quantity of fat and calories as ordinary butter, but they have the advantage of containing a fat that is better for your heart.

–   For most cake recipes, you can reduce the sugar content by half, for example Victoria sandwich, rock cakes, tea breads. As you and your family get used to a less sweet taste you may find that for some recipes, particularly fruit cakes or tea breads, you don't need to add any sugar, but can rely on the dried fruit or even vegetables such as grated carrot or courgette for sweetness, which will also give you extra fibre and minerals such as iron.

–   Using semi-skimmed milk for cooking reduces the fat content of a dish. (Remember that skimmed milk is unsuitable for children under five.)

–   For recipes using mince, there is no need to add extra oil when browning the mince, particularly if using a non-stick pan. Choose lean minced beef where possible. Alternatively, drain off any excess fat after browning.

–   If you do need to use oil in a recipe, try to reduce the amount required and measure with a tablespoon rather than pouring straight from the bottle. Remember that 1 tablespoon of oil has around 100 calories!

–   Choose oils that are high in monounsaturated fat (such as olive or rapeseed oil) or polyunsaturated fat such as corn or sunflower oil.

–   Try reducing the amount of meat used in the recipes, by including more vegetables such as carrots, or pulses such as lentils. This will help to increase the fibre in the dish, give more servings and is also cheaper. A good example is to add a small tin of baked beans to a Spaghetti Bolognese or Shepherd's Pie recipe. (Remember that this will add extra carbohydrate to the total recipe).

USEFUL INGREDIENT MEASURES

Weights

1 oz/25 g	9 oz/250 g
2 oz/50 g	10 oz/275 g
3 oz/75 g	11 oz/300 g
4 oz/100 g	12 oz/350 g
5 oz/150 g	13 oz/375 g
6 oz/175 g	14 oz/400 g
7 oz/200 g	15 oz/425 g
8 oz/225 g	16 oz/450 g

Measuring spoons
½ tsp = 1 x 2.5 ml spoon
1 tsp = 1 x 5 ml spoon
1 dsp = 1 x 10 ml spoon
1 tbsp = 1 x 15 ml spoon

Liquid measures
¼ pint = 150 ml
½ pint = 275 ml
¾ pint = 425 ml
1 pint = 550 ml
2 pint = 1 litre

Useful dimensions
Diameter for cake tins, flan rings, pie plates
6 inch = 15 cm
7 inch = 18 cm
8 inch = 20 cm
9 inch = 23 cm
10 inch = 26 cm
11 inch = 28 cm
12 inch = 30 cm

Oven temperatures

Centigrade	Fahrenheit	Gas
150	300	No 2
160	325	No 3
180	350	No 4
190	375	No 5
200	400	No 6
220	425	No 7
230	450	No 8
240	475	No 9

Diameter for cutter for scones and biscuits
1 inch = 2.5 cm
2 inch = 5 cm
3 inch = 7.5 cm
4 inch = 10 cm
5 inch = 13 cm

Note: When making any of the recipes in this book, only follow one set of measures (ie metric or imperial) as they are not interchangeable.

Eggs

Unless stated, size 3 eggs have been used in the recipes.

Spoon measures

All spoon measures given in this book are level unless otherwise stated.

Starters

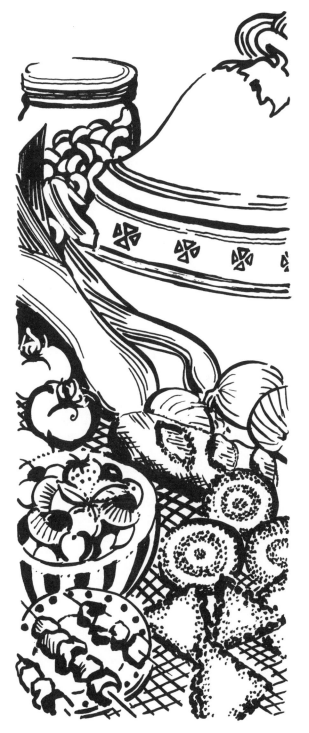

I've included a range of starters from very light dishes such as Chilled Fruit-Filled Melon to more filling soups. The soups could also be used as a light lunch served with fresh crusty bread.

If you don't have time to soak pulses overnight you can use a quick method. Cover the pulses with plenty of boiling rather than cold water and soak for only 2-3 hours or bring the pulses slowly to the boil in a large pan of water. Simmer for 2 minutes and then cover, turn off the heat and soak for only 1 hour.

Black-Eyed Bean and Vegetable Soup

The black-eyed beans, sometimes called black-eyed peas or cowpeas, are an attractive addition with their creamy colour and small black 'eye'. They add a creamy flavour too. Remember if using dried beans to soak overnight before starting this recipe.

1	can (14 oz/400 g) black-eyed beans, drained and rinsed	1
1 tbsp	olive or sunflower oil	15 ml
2	medium onions, peeled and finely diced	2
1	clove garlic, crushed (optional)	1
8 oz	carrots, peeled and finely diced	225 g
1	green pepper, finely diced	1
2	large courgettes, sliced	2
3 pt	boiling vegetable stock, home-made or a cube	1.6 litres
	salt and freshly ground black pepper	
	freshly chopped parsley to garnish	

Heat the oil in a large saucepan and cook the onion until soft. Add the garlic, if using, carrot, green pepper and courgette and cook for a few minutes. Add the stock, seasoning and beans. Stir well. Bring to the boil, cover and simmer gently for 50 minutes until the beans are cooked through. Check seasoning and serve sprinkled with chopped parsley. Serves 4.

PER SERVING	
calories	156
g fat	4
g protein	8
g carbohydrate	22

Leeks are difficult to clean if you want to keep them whole but for a recipe like this, where they are to be puréed, slice lengthways first and then across. The layers will separate out and you can wash them thoroughly in a colander.

Fresh Leek Soup with Stilton

The inspiration for this recipe came from a delicious soup served at a friend's wedding reception. I decided to experiment at home to develop a similar recipe. I think the flavours of leeks and Stilton complement each other well.

1 tbsp	olive or corn oil	15 ml
1	large onion, peeled and chopped	1
1½ lb	leeks, sliced	675 g
1 tbsp	plain flour	15 ml
1½ pt	vegetable or chicken stock	825 ml
3 tbsp	dry white wine	45 ml
	salt and freshly ground black pepper	
2 oz	blue Stilton cheese, crumbled	50 g
¼ pt	semi-skimmed milk	150 ml

Heat the oil in a heavy-based pan and add the onion and leeks. Cook for 5 minutes until softened, but not coloured. Stir in the flour and cook for 1 minute. Remove the pan from the heat and gradually stir in the stock, wine and seasoning. Return the pan to the heat and bring to the boil, stirring constantly. Reduce the heat and simmer gently, uncovered, for 20-30 minutes.

Process in a food processor or liquidiser until smooth. Return to the rinsed-out pan and add the Stilton and milk. Heat gently, stirring constantly, until melted. Season to taste. Serve hot with a wholemeal or Granary roll. Serves 4.

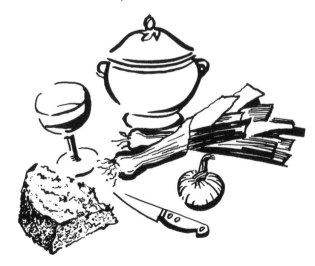

PER SERVING	
calories	176
g fat	8
g protein	8
g carbohydrate	15

Greek Supper Menu
*Quick Chick Pea Dip (page 24)
served with pitta bread fingers
Low-Fat Pastitsio (page 93)
served with Greek Islands'
Crunchy Salad (page 58) as a
side salad
Fresh fruit for dessert or
Raspberry Ice (page 176)*

Quick Chick Pea Dip

On returning from a holiday in Crete we held a 'Greek night' for friends where I made this dish. It is simple to make and will impress your guests who will believe you bought it! Tahini is a sesame paste which is available from health food shops, delicatessens and many supermarkets. Use small lemons otherwise they may overpower the flavour of the dip.

1	can (14 oz/400 g) chick peas, drained	1
2	small lemons, juice of	2
4 tbsp	tahini paste	60 ml
3	cloves garlic, crushed	3
pinch	cayenne pepper	pinch
1 tbsp	chopped fresh parsley to garnish	15 ml

Place the chick peas in a food processor or liquidiser with the lemon juice. Blend until smooth. Add the tahini, garlic and cayenne pepper and mix until blended. Sprinkle with parsley and chill before serving. Serve with warm pitta bread.
Serves 4.

PER SERVING	
calories	210
g fat	13
g protein	9
g carbohydrate	13

Kidney beans are a colourful addition to a soup. Canned ones are easy and quick to use but if you decide to use dried kidney beans, red or black, it is most important they are cooked properly. They must be boiled hard for 10-15 minutes before reducing the heat and simmering until tender. They contain a toxin that is destroyed by boiling but can be dangerous if this is not done.

Italian Red Bean and Pasta Soup

A filling, low-fat soup, also suitable for a lunch or light supper. You can use any pasta for this soup but look for small pasta shapes, made specially for soup. They come in a variety of designs, some of which are particularly appealing to children.

2 tsp	olive or sunflower oil	10 ml
1	medium onion, finely diced	1
4	sticks celery, sliced	4
1/2 tsp	dried thyme	2.5 ml
1	can (7 oz/200 g) red kidney beans, rinsed and drained	1
1	can (14 oz/400 g) chopped tomatoes	1
1 1/4 pt	vegetable stock	700 ml
	salt and freshly ground black pepper	
2 oz	dried pasta shapes	50 g

Heat the oil in a large saucepan and cook the onion, celery and thyme for 4-5 minutes, over a moderate heat, stirring occasionally. Add the beans, tomatoes, stock and seasoning. Bring to the boil, cover and simmer gently for 30 minutes. Add the pasta and cook for a further 10-12 minutes until the pasta is tender. Serve hot with fresh Wholemeal or Granary bread. Serves 2.

PER SERVING	
calories	263
g fat	4
g protein	12
g carbohydrate	46

This dip is delicious with potato skins. See page 31 for a Crispy Potato skins recipe and serve as an alternative to the tomato dip recipe given there.

Quick Tomato Salsa

This dish is as colourful as the Puerto Rican big-band dance music from which it takes its name. You can vary the amount of Tabasco sauce according to how spicy you like your food. Salsa is a popular Mexican dish usually served with tortilla chips or potato skins.

1	can (14 oz/400 g) chopped tomatoes, drained	1
1	small onion, very finely chopped	1
2	cloves garlic, crushed	2
1 tbsp	white wine vinegar	15 ml
1 tbsp	tomato purée	15 ml
1 tbsp	lemon juice	15 ml
½ tsp	Tabasco sauce	2.5 ml
	freshly ground black pepper	

Combine all the ingredients together in a small bowl. Cover and chill until required. Serve with tortilla chips. Serves 6.

PER SERVING	
calories	17
g fat	0
g protein	1
g carbohydrate	4

Right:
Italian Red Bean and Pasta Soup (page 25)

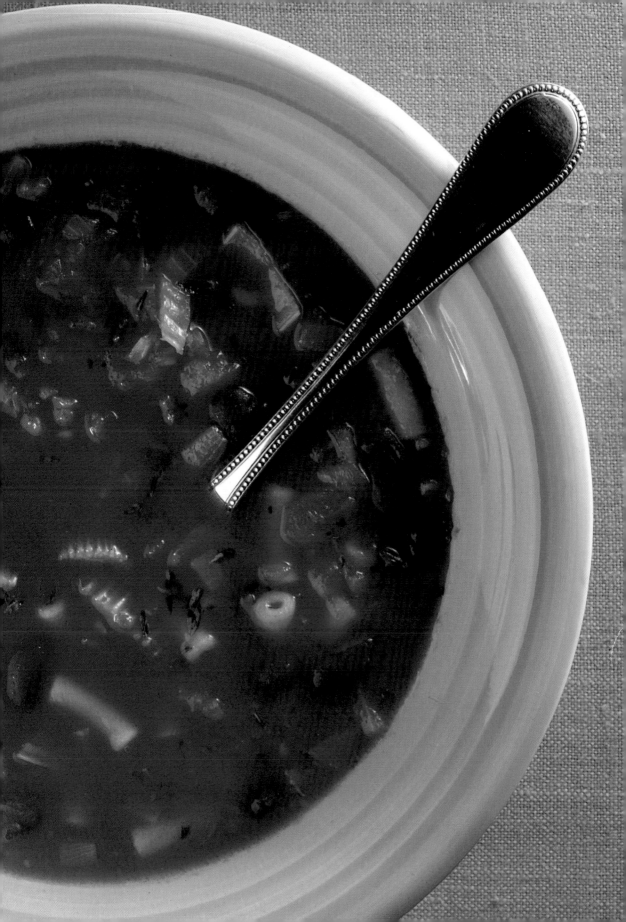

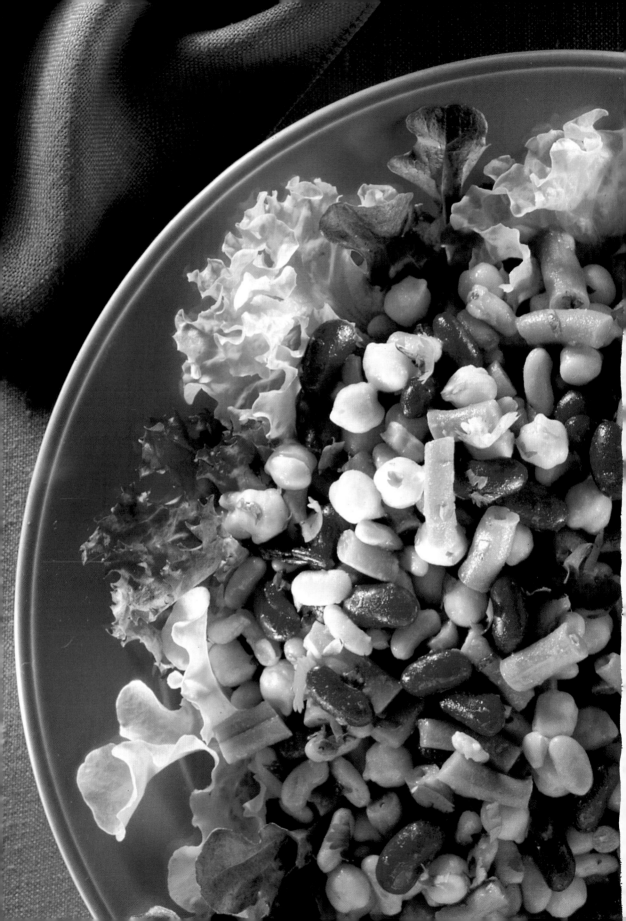

Serve this colourful soup with a vegetable garnish. Have some extra or reserve a little of the tomato, pepper, onion and cucumber and cut into small dice. Sprinkle on top of the soup before serving. It is also delicious served with garlic croûtons.

Low-fat garlic croûtons
Cream a little low-fat spread with a crushed clove of garlic. Spread on to a thick slice of bread. Cut into cubes and put on baking sheet. Bake at 200°C (400°F) Gas Mark 6 for 10 minutes or until crisp and golden.

Chilled Summer Gazpacho

A refreshing chilled soup to serve in the summer with fresh crusty bread. Depending on the capacity of your food processor or liquidiser, you may find it easier to process the vegetables in stages before adding the remaining ingredients to get a smoother result. Do make sure that the soup is thoroughly chilled before serving.

2 lb	ripe red tomatoes, roughly chopped	900 g
1	large onion, roughly chopped	1
1	green pepper, deseeded and chopped	1
1	medium cucumber, chopped	1
3 tbsp	red wine vinegar	45 ml
1 tbsp	olive oil	15 ml
2	cloves garlic, crushed	2
1	jar (20 oz/550 g) Passata (see page 121)	1
	salt and freshly ground black pepper	

Place the tomatoes in a food processor or liquidiser and blend for a few seconds. Add the onion, pepper and cucumber and process until smooth. Finally, add the remaining ingredients and process for a few more seconds. Adjust seasoning to taste, place in a large serving bowl, cover and chill before serving. Serves 6-8.

PER SERVING	
calories	80
g fat	2
g protein	3
g carbohydrate	12

Left:
Easy Green and Red Bean Salad (page 56)

Mulligatawny first became popular in Britain at the end of the eighteenth century when it was brought back to this country by employees of the East India Company after they had been stationed overseas. It was changed for the British cooks and is traditionally seasoned with curry powder quite differently from the spice blends that would have been used in the South Indian original. The word comes from the Tamil words for 'pepper' and 'water'.

Spicy Winter Mulligatawny

A spicy soup for the winter months. Serve with fresh wholemeal or Granary bread. For a vegetarian dish you could easily omit the chicken and use a good vegetable stock without spoiling the flavour.

1 oz	soft margarine	25 g
1	large onion, finely chopped	1
2	cloves garlic, crushed	2
2	sticks celery, sliced	2
8 oz	carrots, peeled and diced	225 g
1-2 tbsp	curry powder	15-30 ml
1 tbsp	plain flour	15 ml
1 tbsp	tomato purée	15 ml
2 pt	hot chicken stock	1 litre
1	medium cooking apple, peeled, cored and diced	1
4 oz	cooked, lean chicken, diced	100 g

Melt the fat in a large saucepan and cook the onion, garlic, celery and carrot for 3-4 minutes until soft. Stir in the curry powder and flour and cook for 1 minute. Stir in the tomato purée and gradually add the stock. Finally, add the apple, bring to the boil and simmer for 20 minutes.

Remove from the heat, and liquidise in a food processor for a few seconds. Return to the saucepan, add the diced chicken and reheat until the chicken is heated through. Serve immediately with fresh wholemeal or Granary bread. Serves 4.

PER SERVING	
calories	144
g fat	6
g protein	7
g carbohydrate	15

Patio Picnic
These tasty satay sticks could
also be served as a summer
main course for a patio lunch
or a picnic. *Serve with
Couscous and Apricot Salad
(page 84) or Red Pepper, Red
Bean and Rice Salad (page 74)
fresh crusty bread and a green
salad. This quantity would
serve 4.*

Spicy Chicken Satay with Creamy Peanut Dip

A delicious starter to nibble. Don't worry if the dip looks
slightly curdled after cooking. Simply allow to cool completely
then beat in the milk. Give the dip a quick stir before serving.

1 lb	skinless and boneless chicken breast fillets	450 g
1	small onion, finely chopped	1
1	clove garlic, crushed	1
2 tbsp	light soy sauce	30 ml
2 tbsp	white wine vinegar	30 ml
1 tsp	olive or sunflower oil	5 ml
1 tsp	mild curry powder	5 ml
1 tsp	chilli powder	5 ml
4 oz	crunchy peanut butter	100 g
7 fl oz	water	200 ml
1 tbsp	skimmed milk	15 ml

Place the chicken between two sheets of greaseproof paper
and flatten with a rolling pin. Cut into 1-inch (2.5-cm) pieces
and place in a shallow container.

Mix the onion and garlic with the soy sauce and vinegar.
Pour over the chicken and toss well. Cover and refrigerate
overnight.

Meanwhile, make the dip. Heat the oil in a small pan.
Add the curry and chilli powder and cook for 30-60 seconds,
stirring. Add the peanut butter and water. Simmer for 2-3
minutes, until thick, stirring constantly. Allow to cool
completely then stir in the milk. Refrigerate until required.

Thread the chicken on to cocktail sticks and place on baking
trays. Cook at 220°C (425°F) Gas Mark 7 for 10-15 minutes
until cooked through, turning halfway through cooking.
Brush with the marinade during cooking. Chill until required.
Serve the chicken pieces cold with the peanut dip.
Serves 4.

PER SERVING	
calories	330
g fat	21
g protein	30
g carbohydrate	5

Suitable for freezing: wrap well in foil. Cook from frozen in a preheated oven at 200°C (400°F) Gas Mark 6 for 40-45 minutes.

Herb and Garlic Bread

I always make my own garlic bread as I find shop bought ones disappointing and also it is more economical to make your own.

4 oz	soft margarine, or butter	100 g
2-3	cloves garlic, crushed	2-3
2 tbsp	chopped fresh parsley	30 ml
2 tbsp	chopped fresh chives	30 ml
1	long French stick, wholemeal if preferred	1

Beat together the soft margarine, or butter, garlic and herbs until evenly mixed. Slice the French stick at 1-inch (2.5-cm) intervals, taking care not to cut completely through the loaf. Spread each slice with the low-fat spread mixture.

Wrap the loaf in foil and bake in a preheated oven at 200°C (400°F) Gas Mark 6 for 20-25 minutes. Serve immediately. Serves 8.

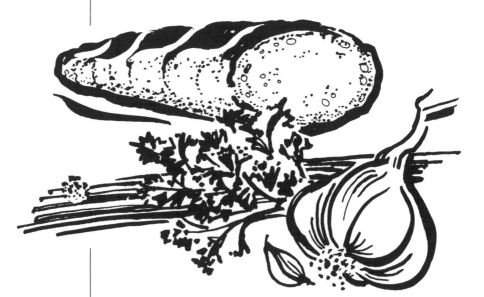

PER SERVING	
calories	194
g fat	11
g protein	4
g carbohydrate	20

Parsley Croquettes
Use the potato you scoop from the skins to make croquettes. Mash with soft margarine and a little skimmed milk. Season with salt and pepper and finely chopped parsley. Form into a roll and cut into 1-inch (2.5-cm) lengths. Chill until firm and coat in egg and breadcrumbs. Freeze until required and then bake on a greased baking sheet at 220°C (425°F) Gas Mark 7 for 15-20 minutes until golden and piping hot.

Crispy Potato Skins with Tomato and Crème Fraîche Dips

Potato skins are popular as a starter and can be easily made for entertaining at home. The dips are also very simple to make. Add the chilli sauce carefully as it can be quite strong. I use a low-fat crème fraîche (French soured cream) which has less than half the fat of ordinary soured cream.

8	small baking potatoes, approximately 4 oz (100 g) each	8
1 tbsp	olive oil	15 ml
	sea salt and freshly ground black pepper	
12 oz	tomatoes, skinned and finely chopped	350 g
2	spring onions, finely chopped	2
1 tbsp	hot chilli sauce	15 ml
5 fl oz	light crème fraîche	150 ml
2 tbsp	fresh chives, chopped	30 ml

Scrub the potatoes thoroughly and dry on kitchen paper. Thread the potatoes on skewers, brush with the oil and sprinkle with salt. Place on an oven shelf in a preheated oven at 200°C (400°F) Gas Mark 6 for 45-55 minutes or until soft.

Meanwhile, make the dips. Mix the tomatoes, onions and chilli sauce together and season with salt and pepper. Place in a serving bowl.

In a separate bowl, mix the crème fraîche and chives together and season to taste. Cover the dips and chill.

Remove the potatoes from the oven and cut in half lengthways. Scoop out the flesh, leaving a layer of potato about 1/2-inch (1-cm) thick on the skin. Cut each skin in half lengthways. Place the skins on a baking tray and return to the oven for 5-10 minutes. Sprinkle with a little extra salt if desired, and serve hot with the dips. Serves 4.

PER SERVING	
calories	292
g fat	8
g protein	7
g carbohydrate	51

Dried beans and peas have the moisture removed to preserve them but they do continue to dry out during storage so the longer they have been stored the longer soaking they will need. It is therefore a good idea to choose pulses from a supplier that has a rapid turnover.

Yellow Split Pea Soup

Split peas do not need soaking overnight as most dried beans do. However, they should be cooked in boiling water for 10 minutes before using in a recipe. This soup would also make a nourishing and filling lunch served with crusty bread.

8 oz	yellow split peas	225 g
1½ pt	vegetable stock	825 ml
1	large onion, finely chopped	1
1	clove garlic, crushed	1
2	carrots, peeled and finely diced	2
1	stick celery, chopped	1
1	can (14 oz/400 g) chopped tomatoes	1
	salt and freshly ground black pepper	

Rinse the split peas in cold water and then drain. Place in a saucepan with plenty of cold unsalted water. Bring to the boil and boil fast for 10 minutes. Drain, rinse and drain again. Return to the pan and add the remaining ingredients. Bring to the boil, cover and simmer for 40-45 minutes or until the peas are soft. Allow to cool, then purée in a liquidiser or food processor. Season well. Reheat gently before serving. Serve with a wholemeal or Granary roll. Serves 6.

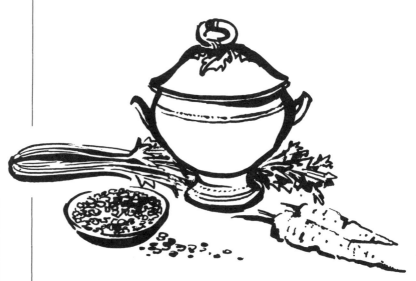

PER SERVING	
calories	143
g fat	1
g protein	10
g carbohydrate	25

Pearl barley is an excellent addition to vegetable soups. It has an interesting texture and flavour but even more importantly, as a grain, the protein it contains adds to the vegetable protein to make a complete protein. The body can use this type much more efficiently than the protein it could get from the vegetables and grains if they were served on their own.

Hearty Winter Vegetable Soup

A nourishing soup which makes use of fresh vegetables in season. It would be ideal for a low-calorie lunch, served with wholemeal or Granary bread.

1 tbsp	olive or sunflower oil	15 ml
1	large onion, finely chopped	1
1	medium swede, cubed	1
2	large carrots, diced	2
1	medium turnip, diced	1
2	leeks, sliced	2
3 oz	pearl barley	75 g
1 tsp	mixed dried herbs	5 ml
2 pt	hot vegetable stock	1 litre
	salt and freshly ground black pepper	
2 tbsp	chopped fresh parsley	30 ml

Heat the oil in a large saucepan, add the vegetables, cover and cook for 5 minutes until soft. Add the barley and cook for 2-3 minutes.

Stir in the herbs, stock and seasoning to taste. Bring to the boil, cover and simmer for 45 minutes until the vegetables are tender. Adjust seasoning and serve sprinkled with chopped fresh parsley. Serve with wholemeal or Granary bread. Serves 4.

PER SERVING	
calories	156
g fat	4
g protein	3
g carbohydrate	28

Ogen and galia melons both have a green flesh. The skin of a galia melon turns from green to a yellowish brown when ripe. A ripe melon will yield a little at the flower end (opposite end to the stalk) but the best way to tell if a melon of this type is ripe is to smell it. There should be a sweet, heady musky perfume from a ripe fruit.

PER SERVING	
calories	70
g fat	0
g protein	2
g carbohydrate	16

For most small crackers, 5 will give approximately 10 g of carbohydrate or you could offer celery sticks to dip in as an alternative.

PER SERVING	
calories	124
g fat	11
g protein	4
g carbohydrate	0

Chilled Fruit-Filled Melon

These attractive fruit-filled melon halves make a light refreshing start to a special meal and are a good way of introducing some extra fruit into your diet.

3	ogen or galia melons	3
2	medium grapefruits	2
1	orange	1
5 oz	frozen raspberries, defrosted and drained	150 g
1	lime, grated rind and juice	1
	a little caster sugar (optional)	
	sprigs of fresh mint to garnish	

Cut the melons in half and discard the seeds. Scoop out a little of the flesh from the centre of each half with a melon baller and place in a bowl. Peel and segment the grapefruits and orange, retaining the juice. Cut the segments in half and place in the bowl, together with the juice and raspberries. Divide the fruit among the melon halves. Sprinkle with a little lime juice, the grated rind and sweetener if using. Refrigerate and serve chilled. Finish each half with a mint sprig. Serves 6.

Quick and Easy Mackerel Pâté

Give your heart a boost with this simple oily-fish spread full of health giving omega-3 fatty acids. As mackerel has quite a strong taste, you only need to use a small amount for each cracker.

8 oz	smoked mackerel fillet, skinned and flaked	225 g
1	carton (7 oz/200 g) reduced-fat soft cheese	1
	a dash of Tabasco sauce	
1-2 tsp	lemon juice	5-10 ml
	freshly ground black pepper	
	lemon slices and parsley to garnish	

Place all the ingredients in a blender or food processor and process until smooth. Season to taste. Chill until required. Serve spread on small crackers and garnish with a little chopped cucumber, red or green peppers or olives. Serves 10.

Little nibbles like these that are easy to pick up are great for starters at a barbecue party. They can be made well in advance and just popped in the oven at the last minute. They are not competing for space on the barbecue and with such tasty morsels guests won't mind the wait while the main course cooks.

Barbecue Party
Cheese and Spinach Filo Triangles (page 35)
Marinated Monkfish Brochettes (page 53) and/or
Marinated Lamb and Rosemary Kebabs (page 97)
Red Pepper, Red Bean and Rice Salad (page 74)
Low-Cal Coleslaw (page 75)
Herb and Garlic Bread (page 30)
Chocolate and Strawberry Roulade (page 179)

Cheese and Spinach Filo Triangles

These triangles look very impressive, yet are fairly simple to make. They look similar to samosas but as they are cooked in the oven rather than fried, they are lower in both fat and calories.

1 lb	frozen chopped spinach, thawed	450 g
1	carton (7 oz/200 g) reduced-fat soft cheese	1
1	clove garlic, crushed	1
1/4 tsp	grated nutmeg	1.25 ml
	grated rind of half a lemon	
	salt and freshly ground black pepper	
6	sheets filo pastry, thawed if frozen	6
2 oz	soft margarine, melted	50 g

Cook the spinach in a saucepan over a gentle heat for approximately 10 minutes, stirring occasionally. Press in a sieve to drain off any remaining water and set aside to cool. Place the soft cheese, garlic, nutmeg and grated lemon rind in a bowl. Season to taste. Beat in the spinach and mix thoroughly. Keep the filo pastry under a damp tea towel while working. Brush one pastry sheet at a time with a little melted fat and cut each strip lengthways into 3 pieces.

Place a heaped teaspoonful of cheese mixture at one end. Fold the pastry over diagonally and keep folding until you reach the end. Continue until all the pastry sheets and filling have been used. Place the triangles on lightly greased baking sheets and brush the tops with the remaining melted fat.

Place in a preheated oven and cook at 200°C (400°F) Gas Mark 6 for approximately 8-10 minutes or until golden brown. Serve hot. Makes approximately 24.

PER TRIANGLE	
calories	41
g fat	4
g protein	1
g carbohydrate	4

Late Summer Celebration Lunch

Watercress and Smoked Salmon Roulade (page 36) served with thin slices of crisp wholemeal toast Creamy Leek and Ham Tart (page 91) served with boiled new potatoes and a green salad or freshly cooked broccoli. Clafouti (page 180) made with small, halved plums if cherries are unavailable.

Watercress and Smoked Salmon Roulade

This makes a delicious light start to a meal. Serve with a salad garnish and thin slices of wholemeal bread. Watercress is very rich in vitamin C, providing 103% of the recommended daily allowance per 100 g.

1	5 oz (150 g) bunch watercress	1
5 oz	reduced-fat soft cheese	150 g
1 tbsp	chopped fresh chives	15 ml
1	clove garlic, crushed	1
1 tsp	lemon juice	5 ml
	freshly ground pepper	
8 oz	smoked salmon	225 g
1	lemon, cut into wedges	1

Reserving a few sprigs for garnish, remove the stalks from the watercress and roughly chop the remainder. Place the watercress, soft cheese, chives, garlic, and lemon juice in a food processor or liquidiser and blend for a few seconds. Season liberally with pepper and process until combined. Lay the pieces of salmon on a sheet of greaseproof paper to form a rectangle approximately 12 x 8 inch (30 x 20 cm). Spread the soft cheese mixture over the salmon, then carefully roll into a thin sausage, lengthways, using the paper to help you. Cover and refrigerate overnight.

Cut the salmon roll into thin slices and serve immediately garnished with lemon wedges, sprigs of watercress and salad vegetables. Serves 4.

PER SERVING	
calories	170
g fat	12
g protein	16
g carbohydrate	0

Fish

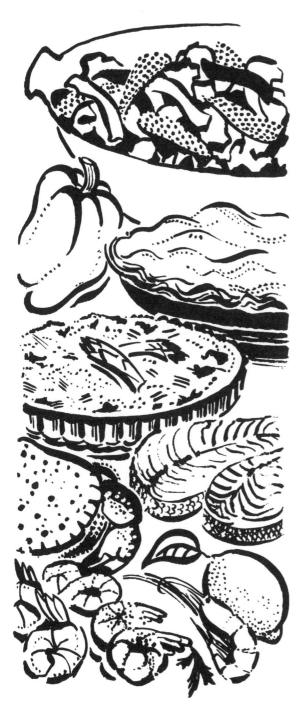

Fish doesn't appear to be high on the agenda of most people in the UK, but it is a food we should all try to eat more frequently. Many people are often put off by the 'fiddly' preparation of fish but these days it could almost be referred to as a convenience food, since most fishmongers or supermarkets can clean and fillet fish for you so that it is ready to use in a recipe. Oily fish such as mackerel, sardines and herring are particularly valuable in the diet as they contain omega-3 fatty acids which appear to have some unique way of protecting against heart disease. Oily fish is also particularly rich in vitamins A and D.

Fresh root ginger is becoming increasingly popular. It is available from all good greengrocers and supermarket fresh produce counters.
It keeps well in the fridge. Store in a plastic bag to prevent drying out.

Oriental Fish Parcels with Ginger and Coriander

A delicious and unusual way of serving mackerel. Serve with noodles and finely shredded vegetables.

4	fresh mackerel, cleaned and filleted	4
1	leek, trimmed and finely sliced	1
1	medium carrot, trimmed and cut into very fine sticks	1
1	courgette, trimmed and cut into very fine sticks	1
1-inch	piece fresh ginger, peeled and grated	2.5-cm
4 tbsp	freshly chopped coriander	60 ml
	salt and freshly ground black pepper	
2 tbsp	light soy sauce	30 ml
1	clove garlic, crushed	1
4 tbsp	dry white wine	60 ml

Cut 4 rectangles of baking parchment or foil large enough to wrap around each fish. Place a mackerel in the centre of each sheet. Arrange the leek, carrot, courgette, ginger and coriander on top of each fish. Season well.

Mix together the soy sauce, garlic and wine and spoon over the fish. Seal each parcel tightly and place on a large baking tray.

Cook in a preheated oven at 200°C (400°F) Gas Mark 6 for 30 minutes or until the fish flakes easily. Serves 4.

PER SERVING	
calories	471
g fat	33
g protein	40
g carbohydrate	3

Midweek Supper for 4
Quick and easy to prepare after a hard day. While the main course is in the oven, you can sit down with your feet up and unwind because the dessert takes just seconds to put together.

Oven-Baked Mushrooms and Cod Crumble (page 39) served with frozen mixed vegetables and jacket potatoes.
Cheat's Cheesecake (page 157).

Oven-Baked Mushroom and Cod Crumble

Porridge oats make a nice crumble topping and are also a good source of soluble fibre which evidence suggests can improve blood glucose (sugar) control. The mushrooms can be replaced by peas or carrots if you like which will also add more colour to the dish.

1½ lb	cod fillets, thawed if frozen, skin removed and boned	675 g
1	medium onion, finely chopped	1
4 oz	mushrooms, sliced	100 g
	salt and freshly ground black pepper	
1	can (10 oz/295 g) mushroom soup	1
3 oz	porridge oats	75 g
1 oz	plain wholemeal flour	25 g
1 tsp	dry mustard	5 ml
2 oz	soft margarine	50 g

Place the cod in a shallow ovenproof dish. Sprinkle the onion and mushrooms over the fish and season to taste. Pour the soup over to cover. Place the oats, flour and mustard in a bowl and rub in the margarine until the mixture resembles breadcrumbs. Sprinkle over the cod mixture. Place in a preheated oven at 190°C (375°F) Gas Mark 5 for 40-50 minutes or until the cod flakes. Serve with freshly cooked vegetables. Serves 4.

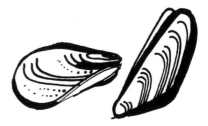

PER SERVING	
calories	355
g fat	15
g protein	33
g carbohydrate	21

Choose tuna packed in water rather than oil to reduce the fat content and calories. If you drain oil-packed tuna you drain away 15-25% of the health-giving omega-3 fatty acids that leach from the fish into the oil. Draining water-packed tuna loses only about 3% of these beneficial fatty acids.

Red Pepper, Basil and Tuna Pasta Salad

Serve with a mixed vegetable or green salad.

2	cans (7 oz/200 g) tuna in water, drained	2
10 oz	pasta twists	275 g
4 oz	French beans, trimmed and sliced	100 g
1	red pepper, deseeded and diced	1
2 tbsp	fresh chopped basil	30 ml
1½ oz	black olives, halved	40 g
4 tbsp	olive oil	60 ml
½ tsp	wholegrain mustard	2.5 ml
2 tbsp	white wine vinegar	30 ml
1	clove garlic, crushed (optional)	1

Flake the tuna and place in a large serving bowl. Cook the pasta in boiling salted water according to the packet instructions, for 8-10 minutes or until al dente. Cool under cold running water and drain well. Meanwhile, cook the French beans and red pepper in lightly salted boiling water for 2-3 minutes until tender. Drain and refresh in cold water. Add to the tuna with the pasta, basil and olives. Chill for 1 hour. Shake the remaining ingredients in a screw-top jar. Toss the salad in the dressing and serve. Serves 4.

PER SERVING	
calories	495
g fat	18
g protein	31
g carbohydrate	55

Garam Masala is a blend of spices rather than just one spice. It is available ready mixed in all good supermarkets and grocers but it is possible to blend your own to complement different dishes. Dry roast the whole spices in a pan and then grind to a powder or mix the ready ground spices. For a fish dish ginger, coriander, cardamom, cumin and dill seeds make a nice combination.

Spicy Tomato and Coconut Fish Curry

This is a delicious way to serve fish as white fish absorbs the curry flavours so well. I find it spicy enough, but my husband prefers a stronger and hotter flavour, so sometimes I add an extra chilli and more garam masala.

2 tbsp	olive or corn oil	30 ml
1	onion, finely chopped	1
2	cloves garlic, crushed	2
1	small green chilli, deseeded, and finely chopped	1
1 tsp	garam masala	5 ml
1 tsp	ground cumin	5 ml
1 tbsp	tomato purée	15 ml
1 tbsp	desiccated coconut	15 ml
1/2 pt	fish stock	275 ml
8 oz	peeled prawns, thawed if frozen	225 g
1 lb	cod fillet, skinned and cubed	450 g
3 oz	frozen peas	75 g
	salt and freshly ground black pepper	

Heat the oil in a large frying pan or wok and stir in the onion, garlic and chilli. Cook for 2-3 minutes, stirring constantly. Stir in the garam masala and cumin. Cook for 2 minutes. Add the tomato purée, coconut and stock and bring to the boil. Reduce the heat and add the prawns, cod, peas and salt and pepper. Half cover and simmer for 10-15 minutes. Serve immediately with freshly cooked brown rice. Serves 4.

PER SERVING	
calories	259
g fat	12
g protein	34
g carbohydrate	5

Midsummer Dinner Party
*Spicy Chicken Satay with Creamy Peanut Dip (page 29) served with pitta bread fingers or French bread
Creamy Crab and Red Pepper Tart (page 42) served with new potatoes and a green salad.
Summer Fruit Layers (page 166) served with thin wafer biscuits*

Creamy Crab and Red Pepper Tart

Crab meat has a 'meaty' texture which makes the tart very filling. You could also use tuna for this recipe as it has a similar texture.

6 oz	plain flour	175 g
3 oz	soft margarine	75 g
1 tbsp	olive or sunflower oil	15 ml
1	small onion, finely diced	1
1	red pepper, deseeded and diced	1
2	cans (6 oz/175 g) white crab meat in brine, drained and flaked	2
3	eggs, beaten	3
8 fl oz	semi-skimmed milk	225 ml
	a pinch of grated nutmeg	
	freshly ground black pepper	

Sieve the flour into a bowl. Rub in the fat until the mixture resembles fine breadcrumbs. Add enough cold water to mix to a soft dough. Chill in the refrigerator for 10 minutes. Roll the pastry out on a lightly floured board and use to line a 9-inch (23-cm) flan tin. Bake blind in a preheated oven at 190°C (375°F) Gas Mark 5 for 10 minutes. Remove the beans and paper and cook for a further 5 minutes.

Meanwhile, heat the oil in a medium saucepan and cook the onion and pepper for 5 minutes or until soft. Scatter over the base of the flan case with the crab meat.

Beat the eggs, milk and nutmeg together and season to taste. Pour into the flan case. Bake in a preheated oven at 180°C (350°F) Gas Mark 4 for 40-50 minutes or until set and golden brown. Serves 8.

PER SERVING	
calories	245
g fat	14
g protein	14
g carbohydrate	16

Tiger prawns are very attractive with their distinctive stripy markings. If you buy them frozen check if they are in a protective ice glaze and if this is included in the weight. Sometimes it can account for almost 50% of the package weight.

Tiger Prawn Jambalaya

I find that fresh tiger prawns can be rather expensive for a weekday meal, but this makes a great informal supper dish for friends. Serve with a side salad.

2 tbsp	olive or sunflower oil	30 ml
2	large onions, finely diced	2
2	red peppers, deseeded and finely diced	2
6	sticks celery, sliced	6
1/2 pt	fish stock	275 ml
1/2 pt	Passata (see page 121)	275 ml
1 tsp	cayenne pepper	5 ml
1 tbsp	chopped fresh thyme	15 ml
2	bay leaves	2
	salt and freshly ground black pepper	
8 oz	rice	225 g
1 lb	fresh raw tiger prawns	450 g
	chopped fresh parsley and lemon wedges to garnish	

Heat the oil in a non-stick frying pan and add the onions, pepper and celery. Cook over a low heat for 5-10 minutes, stirring occasionally, until softened. Stir in the stock, Passata, cayenne pepper, thyme, bay leaves and season to taste. Bring to the boil, cover and simmer for 30 minutes.

Meanwhile, cook the rice according to the packet instructions, until just tender. Drain and keep warm.

Peel the prawns, leaving the tails on. Add the prawns to the sauce mixture and cook for a further 3-5 minutes until the prawns turn pink. Serve with the rice, garnished with parsley and lemon wedges. Serves 4.

PER SERVING	
calories	486
g fat	12
g protein	32
g carbohydrate	65

The fishcakes will freeze. Pack into a rigid container interleaved with pieces of greaseproof paper. Thaw and cook as in the recipe or if you cook from frozen allow 25-30 minutes.

Sweetcorn and Salmon Fishcakes with Yogurt Herb Dressing

The sharp, refreshing yogurt dressing combines well with these salmon fishcakes. Serve with a freshly made salad and new potatoes.

1¹/₂ lb	potatoes, peeled and roughly diced	675 g
2 tbsp	semi-skimmed milk	30 ml
	salt and freshly ground black pepper	
2	cans (7 oz/200 g) pink salmon, bones removed, drained and flaked	2
1	can (7 oz/200 g) sweetcorn with peppers, drained	1
5	spring onions, finely chopped	5
1	small lemon, grated rind and juice	1
1 oz	plain flour	25 g
2 oz	sesame seeds	50 g
10 oz	low-fat natural yogurt	275 g
2 tbsp	chopped fresh chives	30 ml
4-inch	piece cucumber, finely diced	10-cm

Cook the potatoes in boiling salted water for 15 minutes until tender. Drain and mash with the milk and seasoning. Stir in the salmon, sweetcorn, spring onions, half the lemon rind and 2 tablespoons of lemon juice.

Sprinkle a little of the flour on a chopping board. Divide the salmon mixture into 12 and shape into rounds with floured hands. Sprinkle both sides with sesame seeds and gently press into the potato. Chill until required.

Mix the yogurt, chives, remaining lemon rind and cucumber together. Season to taste and chill until required.

Place the fishcakes on lightly greased baking trays and cook in a preheated oven at 190°C (375°F) Gas Mark 5 for 15-20 minutes until golden. Serve hot with the yogurt sauce. Makes 12 fishcakes. Serves 4.

PER SERVING	
calories	459
g fat	16
g protein	31
g carbohydrate	50

July Jollifications
Fresh salmon is probably at its
most reasonable in July. For a
dinner party for 8.

*Chilled Fruit-Filled Melon
(page 34) – use 4 melons and
8 oz (225 g) raspberries for
8 people.
Baked Fresh Salmon and
Spinach in a Light Pastry Case
(page 45) served with new
potatoes, baby carrots and
mange tout
Pineapple and Lemon
Cheesecake (page 159).*

Baked Fresh Salmon and Spinach in a Light Pastry Case

This recipe takes a little time and effort to prepare but is impressive to serve when entertaining.

1/2	lemon, grated rind and juice	1/2
	salt and freshly ground black pepper	
1 tbsp	chopped fresh dill	15 ml
2	fresh salmon fillets approx. 10 oz (275 g) each	2
1 lb 2 oz	puff pastry, thawed if frozen	500 g
12 oz	frozen chopped spinach, thawed and squeezed dry	350 g
4 oz	reduced-fat cream cheese	100 g
4 oz	mushrooms, sliced	100 g
1	egg, beaten	1

Mix the lemon juice and rind, with the black pepper and dill. Rub the mixture into the salmon flesh, and place in a non-metallic dish. Cover and marinate in the fridge for at least 1 hour.

Roll out half the pastry on a lightly floured surface to a rectangle measuring approx. 14 x 6 inches (35 x 15 cm). Place on a large baking sheet and prick all over with a fork.

Bake in a preheated oven at 200°C (400°F) Gas Mark 6 for 12-15 minutes or until golden brown and cooked through. Cool on a wire rack.

Meanwhile, mix the spinach and cream cheese together and season to taste.

Return the cooked pastry to the baking sheet and arrange the salmon fillets on top, skinned side down. Spread the spinach mixture over the fish then layer with the sliced mushrooms.

Roll out the remaining pastry to approximately 15 x 8 inches (38 x 20 cm) and place over the fish and vegetables to completely cover. Trim off any excess pastry. Slash the pastry to form a lattice pattern. Glaze all over with beaten egg. Bake in a preheated oven at 200°C (400°F) Gas Mark 6 for approximately 30-40 minutes or until the fish flakes and the pastry is well risen and golden brown. Serve hot with boiled new potatoes and fresh vegetables. Serves 8-10.

PER SERVING	
calories	338
g fat	24
g protein	13
g carbohydrate	18

Tip. If you buy fresh shellfish, never freeze it. It has almost certainly already been frozen.

Monkfish, Tiger Prawn and Chilli Stir-Fry

Monkfish lends itself well to the robust flavours of this dish. It is one of the more expensive fish but there is no waste. Take care when you handle fresh chillies as they can really irritate the eyes. Make sure that you wash your hands thoroughly after preparing the chillies.

2	garlic cloves, crushed	2
2 tbsp	light soy sauce	30 ml
4 tbsp	dry sherry	60 ml
2 tbsp	lemon juice	30 ml
	freshly ground black pepper	
1	green chilli, deseeded and finely chopped	1
1	bunch spring onions, sliced	1
1 lb	monkfish fillet, cubed	450 g
1 tbsp	olive or sunflower oil	15 ml
4 oz	baby sweetcorn, sliced	100 g
1	green pepper, deseeded and sliced	1
8 oz	cooked, shelled tiger prawns	225 g
2 oz	unsalted cashew nuts	50 g

In a large bowl, mix together the garlic, soy sauce, sherry, lemon juice and pepper. Gently stir in the chilli, onions and monkfish. Cover tightly and leave to marinate in the refrigerator for several hours, turning occasionally.

Drain the marinade and reserve. Heat the oil in a large wok or non-stick frying pan. Add the monkfish mixture and stir-fry over a high heat for 2-3 minutes. Add the baby sweetcorn, green pepper, prawns and cashew nuts and stir-fry for 1-2 minutes. Pour in the marinade, allow to thicken and adjust the seasoning to taste. Serve at once, with freshly cooked rice, or noodles. Serves 4.

PER SERVING	
calories	260
g fat	8
g protein	37
g carbohydrate	5

Tip. A good way to make very thin strips of carrot and courgette is to use a vegetable peeler.

Zesty Lemon Fish Parcels

A quick and attractive way to serve herring. Most fishmongers will clean and fillet the fish for you which saves a lot of time and effort. Serve with boiled new potatoes and freshly cooked vegetables.

1	medium courgette, cut into thin strips	1
1	lemon, thinly sliced	1
1	large carrot, peeled and cut into very thin strips	1
4 oz	button mushrooms, sliced	100 g
4	herrings, filleted	4
4 tbsp	dry white wine	60 ml
	freshly ground black pepper	

Cut four 12 x 18-inch (30 x 45-cm) rectangles from non-stick baking parchment or foil. Divide half the courgette, lemon, carrot and mushrooms among the rectangles. Lay the herring fillets on top and scatter the remaining vegetables and lemon over the top. Sprinkle with the wine and season to taste. Draw up the paper or foil around the fillets and fold the edges to seal. Place on baking sheets. Bake in a preheated oven at 200°C (400°F) Gas Mark 6 for 10-15 minutes. Serve at the table in the parcels for everyone to open. Serves 4.

PER SERVING	
calories	301
g fat	22
g protein	21
g carbohydrate	2

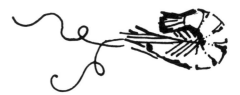

Oven-Baked Fish with Citrus and Coriander Stuffing

Mackerel is one of the oily kinds of fish which we should all be eating more often. This is because the fat found in these fish is mainly of the unsaturated type and there is evidence to suggest that the fatty acids found in fish oils assist in preventing coronary heart disease.

1 tbsp	olive or sunflower oil	15 ml
1	medium onion, finely chopped	1
3 oz	fresh wholemeal breadcrumbs	75 g
3 tbsp	chopped fresh coriander	45 ml
1	size 4 egg, beaten	1
	salt and freshly ground black pepper	
4	fresh mackerel, cleaned and filleted	4
2	lemons, juice and grated rind	2

Heat the oil in a small saucepan and cook the onion over a medium heat for 2-3 minutes until soft. Drain on kitchen paper. Transfer the onion to a medium-sized bowl and stir in the breadcrumbs and coriander. Add the egg, season to taste and mix together well.

Divide the stuffing among the mackerel fillets, pressing it down well. Fold each fillet over along the backbone to enclose the stuffing.

Arrange the fillets in a lightly greased baking dish. Sprinkle with the lemon juice and rind. Cover and bake in a preheated oven at 190°C (375°F) Gas Mark 5 for 20-30 minutes, basting occasionally, until cooked. Serve with new potatoes and freshly cooked vegetables. Serves 4.

Fishermen's Crispy Filo Pie

This is suitable for entertaining and is relatively low in fat. It is also a good source of vitamin A and folic acid. Filo pastry is a healthy option as it is low in fat. You do need to add fat by brushing it on before cooking but less than other pastries and the great advantage is that you can choose the fat you use; from sinful butter to a healthful monounsaturated olive oil.

8 oz	frozen chopped spinach, thawed	225 g
2 oz	rice	50 g
1 lb	smoked haddock fillet	450 g
7 fl oz	skimmed milk	200 ml
2½ oz	soft margarine	65 g
2 tbsp	plain flour	30 ml
3	sheets filo pastry	3
	salt and freshly ground black pepper	

PER SERVING	
calories	464
g fat	33
g protein	35
g carbohydrate	10

Hint. Different makes of filo pastry come in different sizes. For this recipe cut the sheets of filo pastry to the required size. If you have any waste because your sheets are smaller and you have had to use more of them, brush the waste scraps with a little fat and tear them into pieces. Store in the fridge for 2-3 days and use to top pies such as Sichuan Fish Pie (page 51) or Creamy Vegetable Filo Pie (page 77).

Cook the spinach in boiling water for 3 minutes. Drain well and squeeze out the excess liquid. Set aside.

Cook the rice in boiling salted water until tender. Drain well and cool.

In a covered pan, poach the fish in the milk for approximately 10 minutes until just cooked. Strain and reserve the cooking liquor. Flake the fish, discarding the skin and bones.

Melt 1½ oz (40 g) of the margarine in a saucepan. Stir in the flour and cook for 1 minute. Stir in the reserved liquor, bring to the boil and cook for 1-2 minutes or until thickened. Carefully stir in the fish. Season and set aside to cool.

Melt the remaining margarine. Cut one sheet of filo pastry horizontally into 3 equal portions to give rectangles approximately 5 x 7½ inch (12.5 x 19 cm). Place one rectangle on a lightly greased baking sheet. Brush the pastry lightly with the melted fat. Continue layering with the remaining two rectangles. Spoon the rice mixture on to the pastry, leaving a 1-inch (2.5-cm) border all around. Cover the rice with spinach and then top with the fish. Cut the remaining filo pastry sheets in half and place one half on top of the filling. Brush with the fat. Layer with the remaining pastry as before. Seal the edges well and brush the top with the melted fat. Bake in a preheated oven at 200°C (400°F) Gas Mark 6 for approximately 20-30 minutes or until crisp and golden brown. Serve with boiled new potatoes and freshly cooked vegetables. Serves 6.

PER SERVING	
calories	198
g fat	11
g protein	15
g carbohydrate	10

Sweet Pepper, Baby Corn and Smoked Fish Stir-Fry

Mackerel does have a strong flavour which is not to everyone's taste. However, this stir-fry uses lots of fresh vegetables and hence only a small amount of mackerel is required per serving which may persuade any reluctant fish eaters in your household.

1 tbsp	olive or sunflower oil	15 ml
1	small onion, thinly sliced	1
1	clove garlic, crushed	1
1	red pepper, deseeded and sliced	1
1	green pepper, deseeded and sliced	1
4 oz	baby sweetcorn, sliced	100 g
8 oz	skinned smoked mackerel fillet, sliced	225 g
8 oz	beansprouts	225 g
4 tbsp	dry sherry or red wine	60 ml
	freshly ground black pepper	

PER SERVING	
calories	293
g fat	22
g protein	14
g carbohydrate	8

Heat the oil in a large frying pan or wok, and cook the onion and garlic for 2-3 minutes, stirring. Stir in the peppers and baby sweetcorn and cook for a further 2 minutes. Stir in the mackerel and cook for 4 minutes, stirring carefully.

Add the beansprouts, sherry or wine and seasoning and cook for a further 2 minutes. Serve immediately with brown rice or noodles. Serves 4.

Quick-Grilled Salmon with Garlic and Peppercorns

This salmon dish can be prepared in advance and takes very little time to cook, which makes it just perfect for entertaining friends, especially if you are like me and don't like missing out on the conversation while you are busy in the kitchen! Farmed salmon is no more expensive than cod these days but a tail piece is cheaper than steaks.

1	lemon, juice of	1
2	cloves garlic, crushed	2
4 fl oz	dry white wine	100 ml
1 tbsp	crushed mixed peppercorns	15 ml
6	6 oz (175 g) salmon steaks	6
2	lemons, sliced	2

Mix the lemon juice, garlic, wine and peppercorns together. Place the salmon steaks in a shallow dish and pour over the lemon juice mixture. Arrange the lemon slices on top of the steaks, cover and leave to marinate in the refrigerator for 2 hours or overnight.

Remove the lemon slices and grill the salmon steaks under a hot grill for 4-5 minutes each side, basting with the marinade mixture during cooking. Serve garnished with the lemon slices. Serves 6.

PER SERVING	
calories	329
g fat	19
g protein	35
g carbohydrate	0

Suitable for freezing. Thaw and reheat as for the cooking time. Cover with foil if the pastry overbrowns. Don't worry if you have used frozen fish for this dish. You can still freeze it because the fish has been cooked after thawing thus destroying any harmful bacteria and rendering it safe to freeze again. It would, however, not be advisable to refreeze any portion that was left over after it had been reheated.

Sichuan Fish Pie

Many people find white fish has a bland taste, but this recipe shows that fish is excellent served as a spicy dish. Vary the amount of chilli to your taste as the quantity used is quite hot.

1 tbsp	olive or sunflower oil	15 ml
1½ lb	coley or cod fillet, skinned, bones removed and cubed	675 g
1	red pepper, deseeded and sliced	1
1	green pepper, deseeded and sliced	1
2	courgettes, diced	2
2 tbsp	light soy sauce	30 ml
2 tbsp	chilli sauce (or to taste)	30 ml
1	lemon, juice of	1
1-inch	piece fresh root ginger, grated	2.5-cm
¼ pt	fish stock	150 ml
2	sheets filo pastry	2
1 oz	soft margarine, melted	25 g
	salt and freshly ground black pepper	

Heat the oil in a large saucepan, add the fish and vegetables and stir-fry for 5 minutes. Spoon the mixture into a 2-pt (1-litre) ovenproof dish.

Mix together the soy sauce, chilli sauce, lemon juice, ginger and stock. Season and pour over the fish mixture. Brush the pastry sheets with the melted margarine and crumple over the fish. Bake in a preheated oven at 220°C (425°F) Gas Mark 7 for 15-20 minutes or until crisp and golden brown. Serves 4.

PER SERVING	
calories	255
g fat	12
g protein	32
g carbohydrate	6

Spring High Tea for 6
Flaky Salmon and Asparagus Tart (page 52) served with Creamy Curried Potato Salad (page 68) and Tomato, Red Onion and Fresh Chive Salad (page 59) with fresh crusty bread
Apricot Pecan Slice (page 132)

Flaky Salmon and Asparagus Tart

A colourful savoury tart which is particularly suitable for a high tea or buffet. Make this for a late spring treat to have in the garden. Fresh English asparagus is at its best late May and early June.

For the pastry

2oz	plain flour	50 g
2 oz	wholemeal self-raising flour	50 g
3 oz	soft margarine	75 g

For the filling

1	can 7 oz (200 g) salmon in brine, drained	1
6	asparagus tips	6
2	size 2 eggs	2
1/4 pt	skimmed milk	150 ml

Sieve the flours together into a bowl, tipping any bran remaining in the sieve into the bowl. Rub the margarine into the flour until the mixture resembles breadcrumbs. Add enough water to bind to a soft dough. Roll out thinly to line an 8-inch (20-cm) flan dish. Chill for 30 minutes. Flake and bone the salmon and place in the base of the flan dish. Blanch the asparagus tips in boiling salted water for 5 minutes. Drain and arrange on top of the salmon. Beat the eggs and milk together, add seasoning to taste. Pour over the asparagus to fill the pastry case. Bake in a preheated oven at 200°C (400°F) Gas Mark 6 for 35-40 minutes. Serve either hot or cold. Serves 6.

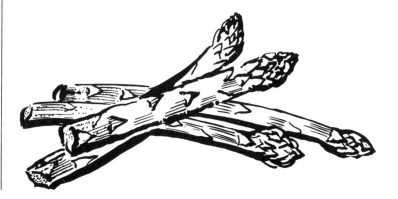

PER SERVING	
calories	208
g fat	12
g protein	12
g carbohydrate	14

Tip. If you use wooden skewers for kebabs, soak them in hot water until they sink before threading the food on to them. This will stop them charring during cooking.

Marinated Monkfish Brochettes

Monkfish is ideal for kebabs as it keeps its shape well when cooked. I find fish kebabs make a nice change when holding a barbecue, or these can be cooked under a grill for a simple supper. Vary the vegetables to suit your family's tastes or to use what you have at hand in the refrigerator.

5 tbsp	olive or sunflower oil	75 ml
1	large lemon, grated rind and juice	1
2	sprigs of thyme	2
2	bay leaves	2
1 tbsp	freshly chopped parsley	15 ml
	salt and freshly ground black pepper	
1½ lb	monkfish, bone removed and cubed	675 g
8 oz	cherry tomatoes	225 g
2	large green peppers, deseeded and cut into bite-sized pieces	2
4 oz	baby mushrooms	100 g
8 oz	shallots	225 g

For the marinade, mix the oil with the lemon rind, juice, herbs and seasoning to taste. Skewer the fish alternately with the vegetables on 8 skewers and place in a shallow dish. Pour the marinade over, cover and chill in the refrigerator for 2 hours, turning occasionally.

Remove the brochettes from the marinade. Place on a barbecue and cook until the fish becomes opaque and the vegetables are lightly browned, turning and basting frequently with the marinade. Alternatively, cook under a preheated grill for 10 minutes. Serve with freshly cooked rice. Serves 4.

PER SERVING	
calories	341
g fat	20
g protein	32
g carbohydrate	9

Summer Lunch for 2
*Fresh Prawn and Herb
Omelette (page 54) served with
Tomato, Red Onion and Fresh
Chive Salad (page 59) and
slices from a warm Granary
Loaf (page 150)
Fresh fruit to finish*

Fresh Herb and Prawn Omelette

This light and tasty omelette is ideal for summer when fresh
herbs are in abundance in the garden or on your windowsill.
If your green fingers fail you, all good supermarkets have
packets of fresh herbs these days and even pots of 'growing
herbs' for you to start your own herb garden. If all else fails,
substitute dried herbs in place of fresh. You will need around
$1/2$ tsp of dried herbs to replace the fresh herbs in the recipe.

4	eggs, beaten	4
	salt and freshly ground black pepper	
2 tbsp	skimmed milk	30 ml
1 tbsp	olive or sunflower oil	15 ml
3 oz	peeled prawns, thawed if frozen	75 g
1 tbsp	fresh chopped herbs such as parsley, tarragon	15 ml

Whisk together the eggs, seasoning and milk. Heat the oil in
a medium-sized non-stick frying pan. When really hot, tip in the
eggs. Cook over a moderate heat until lightly set. Sprinkle the
prawns and herbs over the eggs and cook for 2-3 minutes to
heat through. Fold in half and serve immediately. Serve with
freshly made salad and crusty bread. Serves 2.

PER SERVING	
calories	291
g fat	22
g protein	24
g carbohydrate	0

Vegetarian

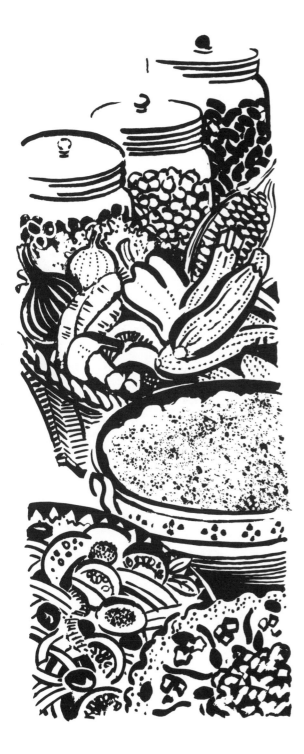

This section includes a variety of main course recipes as well as fresh salads and vegetable side dishes to accompany meals. I have tried to include lots of pulses such as beans and lentils which contain soluble fibre. Soluble fibre can help to control blood glucose levels by slowing down the rate at which sugars in foods get into the blood. It can also help to reduce the amount of cholesterol in the blood. I enjoy vegetarian food and quite often choose the vegetarian option when dining out. I particularly like the spicy recipes in this section and experimenting with different vegetables.

Dressing the beans well in advance allows them to absorb all the flavours but if you dress the salad leaves too far in advance they become too wet and lose their crunch. If you need to display the food in advance such as for a buffet, you can serve the bean salad in a small dish set among the green leaves.

Easy Green and Red Bean Salad

I prefer to use flat leaf parsley for the dressing. It's more distinctly flavoured than curled parsley and can be found in generous bunches in many Asian grocer's shops.

5 oz	French green beans, trimmed and cut in small pieces	150 g
1	can (14 oz/400 g) red kidney beans, rinsed and drained	1
1	can (14 oz/400 g) flageolet beans, rinsed and drained	1
1	can (14 oz/400 g) chick peas, rinsed and drained	1
2 tbsp	fresh parsley, chopped	30 ml
1	lemon, juice only	1
2 tbsp	white wine vinegar	30 ml
5 tbsp	olive oil	75 ml
	freshly ground black pepper	
	lettuce leaves to garnish	

Lightly steam the green beans over boiling water for 5-6 minutes. Drain. Place in a large bowl with the kidney beans, flageolet beans and chick peas and mix well.

In a jar, mix together the parsley, lemon juice, vinegar, olive oil and pepper. Pour over the bean mixture and toss lightly to mix. Chill until required.

Just before serving, place the lettuce leaves around the edge of a large serving dish. Spoon the bean mixture over the leaves and serve. Serves 6-8 as a side salad.

PER SERVING	
calories	301
g fat	15
g protein	13
g carbohydrate	30

The cooked but unfilled choux ring can be frozen. Cool, split horizontally and put a sheet of greaseproof paper between the halves. Pack into a rigid container. Thaw before filling.

Mediterranean Gougère

I've found that ordinary flour gives a better result than wholemeal flour for choux pastry. The small difference in fibre is made up by the vegetables in this recipe. I use a food processor to add the eggs to the choux mixture to obtain a smooth, glossy result. Do use a slotted spoon to spoon the vegetables into the choux ring so that the filling is not too runny.

2½ oz	soft margarine	65 g
7 fl oz	cold water	200 ml
4 oz	plain flour, sifted	100 g
3	eggs, beaten	3
3 oz	cheddar, grated	75 g
1 tbsp	olive or sunflower oil	15 ml
1	small onion, finely diced -	1
2	garlic cloves, crushed	2
1	green pepper, deseeded and diced	1
1	red pepper, deseeded and diced	1
2	small courgettes, sliced	2
1	can (14 oz/400 g) tomatoes, drained	1
1 tbsp	chopped fresh mixed herbs	15 ml
	salt and freshly ground black pepper	

Place the margarine and water in a saucepan and heat gently until the margarine has melted. Bring to the boil, remove from the heat and add the flour all at once. Beat well for 1-2 minutes, or until the mixture forms a ball and leaves the sides of the pan clean. Allow to cool slightly. Gradually add the eggs a little at a time, beating hard until the mixture is smooth, thick and glossy. Beat in half the cheese and season well. Draw an 8-inch (20-cm) circle on a sheet of baking parchment and place on a baking sheet. Spoon or pipe the choux mixture on to the paper to form a circle.

Place in a preheated oven at 220°C (425°F) Gas Mark 7 for 20 minutes. Reduce the heat to 190°C (375°F) Gas Mark 5 and cook for a further 10 minutes or until well risen and golden. Carefully remove the paper and cool on a wire rack.

Meanwhile, heat the oil in a medium-sized saucepan. Cook the onion, and garlic for 2-3 minutes, or until soft, stirring occasionally.

PER SERVING	
calories	285
g fat	20
g protein	10
g carbohydrate	19

Add the peppers, cover and cook over a low heat for 5 minutes. Stir in the courgettes, tomatoes and herbs. Cook, uncovered, for a further 15 minutes, or until the vegetables are tender. Season to taste and remove from the heat.

Split the choux ring in half horizontally. Place the bottom half on a baking sheet. Spoon in the filling and cover with the top of the choux ring. Sprinkle with the remaining cheese and return to the oven for 5 minutes to heat through. Serve immediately with jacket potatoes and freshly cooked vegetables or crusty bread. Serves 6.

Feta cheese is traditionally made from ewe's milk but is often made from cow's milk nowadays. It is usually found vacuum packed in brine in the prepacked cheese counter of good supermarkets and delicatessens.

PER SERVING	
calories	282
g fat	25
g protein	8
g carbohydrate	8

Right:
Courgette, Sweetcorn and Red Pepper Pizza (page 71)

Greek Islands' Crunchy Salad

This is my favourite dish for a simple lunch with crusty bread when holidaying in the Greek islands. It can also be served as a side salad where it will serve 4. If you are watching calories, omit the oil and this will save a total of 200 calories.

1/2	iceberg lettuce, roughly chopped	1/2
1/2	cucumber, diced	1/2
2	beef tomatoes, sliced	2
3 oz	Feta cheese, crumbled	75 g
8	black olives in brine, stoned and drained	8
2 tbsp	olive oil	30 ml
	freshly ground black pepper	

Arrange the lettuce, cucumber, tomatoes, cheese and olives between two serving dishes. Drizzle with the oil and season with black pepper to taste. Serves 2.

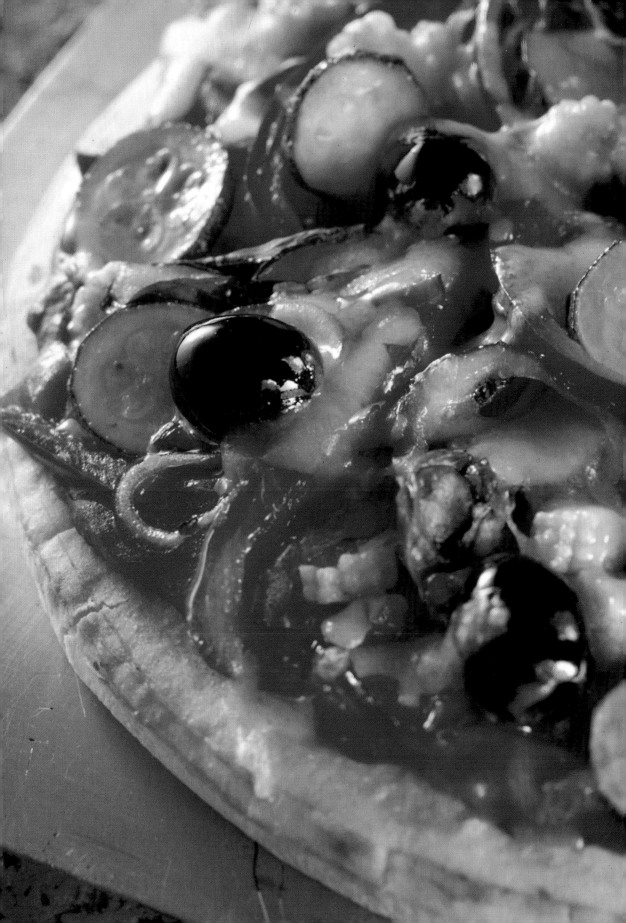

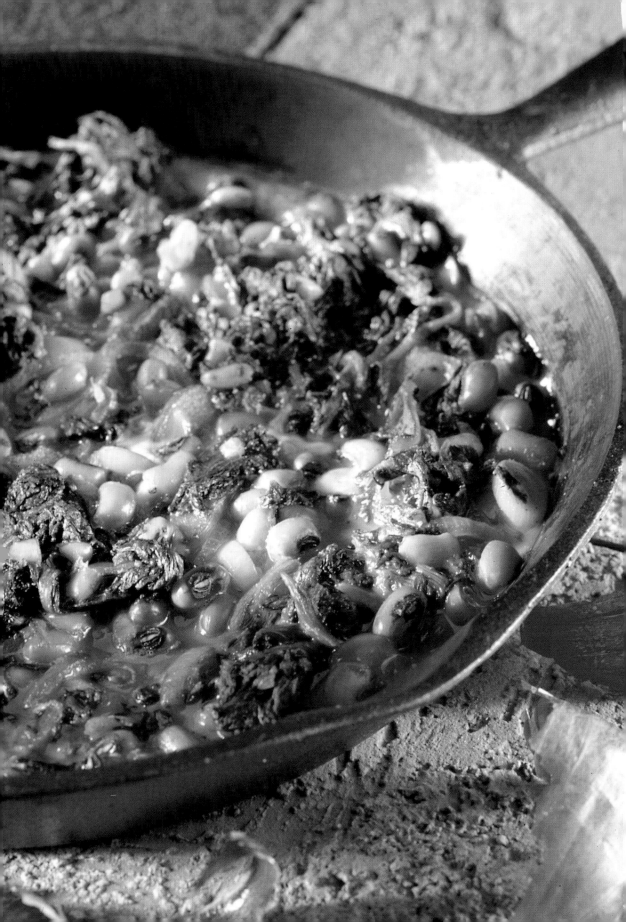

Beef tomatoes are extra large and sometimes irregular in shape. They are usually imported from Holland. They are particularly good in salads because they have a good firm texture. If they are a little lacking in flavour the red onion and full-flavoured dressing in this salad more than make up for it.

Tomato, Red Onion and Fresh Chive Salad

Balsamic vinegar is an intense, rich, sweet-sour vinegar which has become very popular for cooking as well as salads. You can find it in delicatessens and some larger supermarkets.

3 tbsp	olive oil	45 ml
1 tbsp	balsamic vinegar	15 ml
	salt and freshly ground black pepper	
1½ lb	beef tomatoes, sliced	675 g
2	medium red onions, peeled and sliced	2
	finely chopped fresh chives to garnish	

Whisk together the oil and vinegar and add seasoning to taste. Mix together the tomato and onion and toss in the olive oil mixture. Place in a serving bowl and leave to marinate in the refrigerator for 30 minutes before serving. Garnish with chopped fresh chives. Serves 4 as a side salad.

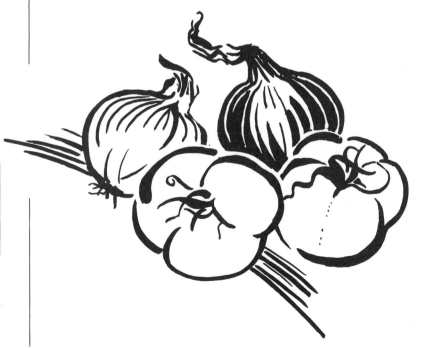

PER SERVING	
calories	141
g fat	12
g protein	2
g carbohydrate	8

Left:
Mexican Black-Eyed Bean and Spinach Tortilla (page 61)

Vary the ingredients with sliced cucumber, strips of green pepper, tiny fresh broad beans or for a treat add a can of drained and quartered artichoke hearts. Artichokes are high in iron and potassium, low in fat and less than 16 calories per 1 oz (25 g).

Light Salad Niçoise

Salad Niçoise can traditionally be quite high in fat. I've reduced the fat content by using canned tuna in brine or water and fat-free French dressing. Both products are readily available in major supermarkets. Serve with fresh crusty bread.

1	iceberg lettuce, finely shredded	1
2	large beef tomatoes, cut into wedges	2
3 oz	cooked and cooled French beans	75 g
6	spring onions, sliced	6
1	garlic clove, crushed	1
4 tbsp	fat-free French dressing	60 ml
2	cans (7 oz/200 g) tuna in water or brine, drained	2
6	anchovy fillets, drained	6
8	stoned black olives in brine, drained	8
4	hard-boiled eggs, shelled and quartered	4

Place the lettuce, tomatoes, beans and spring onions in a serving bowl and toss lightly together. Mix the garlic into the dressing and drizzle half of it over the contents of the bowl. Add the tuna in large chunks. Pat the anchovy fillets dry on kitchen paper and place on top of the tuna with the olives. Drizzle over the remainder of the dressing and finally place the eggs on top of the salad. Serve chilled. Serves 4.

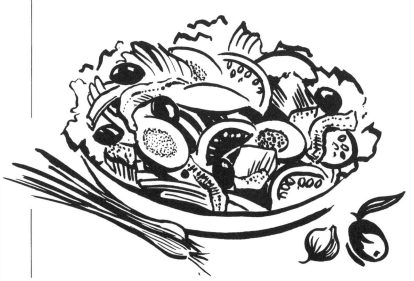

PER SERVING	
calories	246
g fat	11
g protein	33
g carbohydrate	5

Pack a Picnic for 2
*Mexican Black-Eyed Bean and
Spinach Tortilla (page 61)
served with crusty bread,
cherry tomatoes and wedges
of cucumber.
Carrot and Banana Squares
(page 127)
Fresh fruit*

Mexican Black-Eyed Bean and Spinach Tortilla

This is a dish of Spanish origins meaning 'little cake'. It is a great addition to a picnic basket in place of the more usual sandwiches or as a quick dish for a light supper or lunch. Serve with a side salad and fresh crusty bread.

1 tbsp	olive or sunflower oil	15 ml
1	red onion, thinly sliced	1
2	cloves garlic, crushed	2
1 tsp	ground turmeric	5 ml
1	can (14 oz/400 g) black-eyed beans, drained	1
8 oz	frozen leaf spinach, thawed and squeezed dry	225 g
4	eggs	4
	salt and freshly ground black pepper	

   Heat the oil in a large non-stick frying pan and fry the onion, garlic and turmeric for 4-5 minutes. Stir in the beans and spinach.
   Whisk the eggs and seasoning together and stir into the pan to coat the other ingredients thoroughly. Cook for 6-7 minutes until nearly set.
   Place the pan under a hot grill for 2-3 minutes until the omelette is set on top. Cut into wedges and serve hot or cold. Serves 2.

PER SERVING	
calories	515
g fat	23
g protein	36
g carbohydrate	44

Serve with Tomato, Red Onion and Fresh Chive Salad (page 59).

Chick Pea, Apricot and Cashew Nut Pilau

A filling dish which has a lovely combination of textures from the rice, chick peas and cashew nuts. It is a good source of fibre and provides around 6 g per serving. Serve with a light salad such as tomato.

1 tbsp	olive or sunflower oil	15 ml
1	large onion, finely chopped	1
2	cloves garlic, crushed	2
1	large carrot, diced	1
1 tsp	ground cumin	5 ml
1/2 tsp	ground cinnamon	2.5 ml
7 oz	rice	200 g
1 1/4 pt	vegetable stock	700 ml
1	can (14 oz/400 g) chick peas, drained	1
2 oz	ready-to-eat dried apricots, chopped	50 g
3 oz	unsalted cashew nuts	75 g
2 tbsp	chopped fresh coriander	30 ml
	salt and freshly ground black pepper	

Heat the oil in a large non-stick frying pan or wok and cook the onion, garlic and carrot for 5 minutes until soft and golden. Stir in the cumin, cinnamon and rice and cook for 1 minute, stirring.

Stir in the stock, bring to the boil and simmer gently for 40 minutes.

Stir in the chick peas, apricots, cashew nuts, coriander and seasoning. Cook for a further 5-10 minutes, or until all the liquid has been absorbed. Serve hot with a tomato salad. Serves 4.

PER SERVING	
calories	464
g fat	17
g protein	15
g carbohydrate	66

Flageolet beans were developed in Brittany in 1872 by Gabriel Chevrier. They are an essential accompaniment to traditional Breton roast lamb from animals reared on the salt flats around Mont St Michel. This dish could be served as a vegetable accompaniment to plainly cooked lamb in which case it would serve 6.

Flageolet Bean and Mushroom Korma

Flageolet beans are a green kidney bean that are useful to keep on hand in the kitchen. They are delicious just heated up as a vegetable with plain roasted meats and combine well with mushrooms to make this creamy curry.

1 tbsp	olive or sunflower oil	15 ml
1	red onion, chopped	1
8 oz	button mushrooms, quartered	225 g
2	cloves garlic, crushed	2
1-inch	piece fresh root ginger, peeled and grated	2.5-cm
1/4 pt	vegetable stock	150 ml
1	can (14 oz/400 g) flageolet beans, drained	1
1 tbsp	mild curry paste	15 ml
1 tsp	ground coriander	5 ml
	salt and freshly ground black pepper	
2 oz	unsalted cashew nuts	50 g
1	carton (5 oz/150 g) low-fat natural yogurt	1

Heat the oil in a saucepan and cook the onion, mushrooms, garlic and ginger for 5 minutes, stirring. Add the stock, flageolet beans, curry paste, coriander and season to taste. Bring to the boil, cover and simmer for 20 minutes. Add the cashew nuts and cook for 5 minutes. Stir in the yogurt, heat through and serve immediately. Serve with freshly cooked brown rice. Serves 2-3.

PER SERVING	
calories	432
g fat	22
g protein	22
g carbohydrate	38

Suitable for freezing. Thaw completely and then reheat in a saucepan. Simmer for 10 minutes or until piping hot, adding a little extra water or stock if the mixture becomes too dry.

Spicy Cajun Casserole

A filling casserole with a spicy punch. The heat of the chilli really brings out the sweetness of the root vegetables. Serve as a main meal with fresh crusty bread or alternatively, serve in smaller portions as a side vegetable.

1 tbsp	olive or sunflower oil	15 ml
2	medium onions, finely diced	2
2	cloves garlic, crushed	2
3	small carrots, sliced	3
8 oz	parsnips, diced	225 g
8 oz	button mushrooms, halved	225 g
1	green pepper, deseeded and chopped	1
1-2 tsp	chilli powder	5-10 ml
1 tbsp	tomato purée	15 ml
3/4 pt	boiling vegetable stock	275 ml
1	can (14 oz/400 g) tomatoes	1
1	can (14 oz/400 g) black-eyed beans, drained	1
2 tsp	dried mixed herbs	10 ml
	a few drops Tabasco sauce	

Heat the oil in a large saucepan. Add the onion and garlic and cook for 2 to 3 minutes, stirring. Add the carrot, parsnip, mushrooms and pepper and cook for a further 5 minutes, stirring occasionally. Stir in the chilli powder and tomato purée and gradually add the stock. Add the remaining ingredients and bring to the boil. Cover and simmer for 40-50 minutes until tender. Serve with jacket potatoes or crusty bread. Serves 4-6.

PER SERVING	
calories	230
g fat	6
g protein	11
g carbohydrate	36

Suitable for freezing.
Freeze before baking and then
thaw and bake as in the recipe.

Black-Eyed Bean Crumble

I make this crumble topping, using a food processor. I make the breadcrumbs first, add the parsley and diced cheese and then process the mixture for a few seconds to obtain a fine crumble.

1 tbsp	olive or sunflower oil	15 ml
2	cloves garlic, crushed	2
1	leek, sliced	1
3	carrots, diced	3
1	parsnip, diced	1
3	sticks celery, chopped	3
2 tsp	paprika	10 ml
1 tsp	oregano	5 ml
1	can (14 oz/400 g) chopped tomatoes	1
1 tbsp	tomato purée	15 ml
1/4 pt	vegetable stock	150 ml
	salt and freshly ground black pepper	
1	can (14 oz/400 g) black-eyed beans, drained	1
3 oz	fresh wholemeal breadcrumbs	75 g
2 tbsp	chopped fresh parsley	30 ml
1 oz	cheddar, grated	25 g

Heat the oil in a large non-stick saucepan. Add the garlic and leek and cook for 1-2 minutes, stirring. Add the remaining vegetables and stir well. Stir in the paprika, oregano, tomatoes, tomato purée, stock and salt and pepper.

Bring to the boil, cover and simmer for 20-25 minutes until the vegetables are tender, but not soft. Stir in the drained beans and turn into a large ovenproof dish.

Mix together the breadcrumbs, parsley and cheese and season to taste. Sprinkle over the vegetable mixture.

Bake in a preheated oven at 200°C (400°F) Gas Mark 6 for 15-20 minutes, until golden brown. Serve with freshly cooked vegetables and crusty bread or potatoes. Serves 4.

PER SERVING	
calories	271
g fat	7
g protein	14
g carbohydrate	40

For non-vegetarians serve with warm slices of Cheese and Bacon Loaf (page 148).

Lentil and Root Vegetable Hotpot

Lentils are a good source of soluble fibre and provide the base for this filling and nutritious supper dish. Lentils do not require soaking before cooking as other pulses do, however it is important that they are boiled rapidly for 10 minutes as instructed below, before adding to the hotpot.

8 oz	red lentils	225 g
1 tbsp	olive or sunflower oil	15 ml
1	onion, finely diced	1
2	cloves garlic, crushed	2
2	carrots, finely diced	2
1	small swede, cubed	1
3	sticks celery, sliced	3
7 fl oz	Passata (see page 121)	200 ml
1/2 tsp	dried oregano	2.5 ml
1/2 pt	hot vegetable stock	275 ml
	salt and freshly ground black pepper	

Cook the lentils in boiling salted water for 10 minutes. Drain and rinse thoroughly.

Heat the oil in a large saucepan and cook the onion and garlic for 5 minutes until soft. Add the carrots, swede and celery and cook for 1-2 minutes stirring occasionally. Add the lentils and the remaining ingredients, bring to the boil, and simmer for 30-40 minutes, or until the vegetables are tender. Ladle into warmed bowls and serve with fresh crusty bread or warmed pitta bread. Serves 4.

PER SERVING	
calories	241
g fat	5
g protein	14
g carbohydrate	38

The word 'Primavera' is added to a dish to mean with fresh spring vegetables, presumably from the word 'primeurs' meaning early forced vegetable and fruit.

Spring Lunch
Quick Tomato Salsa with tortilla chips (page 26) Risotto Primavera (page 67) served with a crisp salad of finely shredded spring greens. Rhubarb and Ginger Fool (page 161)

Risotto Primavera

This recipe is high in starchy carbohydrate and low in fat. For a non-vegetarian meal, you could add chopped cooked meat such as chicken, when adding the vegetables.

1 tbsp	olive or sunflower oil	15 ml
1	onion, finely chopped	1
2	carrots, diced	2
2	medium courgettes, diced	2
4 oz	baby sweetcorn, sliced	100 g
3	sticks celery, sliced	3
12 oz	rice	350 g
2 tsp	dried mixed herbs	10 ml
2 pt	hot vegetable stock	1 litre
1	beef tomato, skinned, and chopped	1
	salt and freshly ground black pepper	
1 tbsp	chopped fresh parsley	15 ml

Heat the oil in a heavy-based pan. Cook the onion, carrot, courgette, sweetcorn and celery for 5 minutes until just soft. Stir in the rice and herbs and cook for 1-2 minutes, stirring continuously.

Gradually stir in the stock, season, cover and cook for 45-50 minutes, or until all the stock has been absorbed. Add the tomato and cook for 5 minutes. Season well and serve hot, garnished with chopped fresh parsley. Serve with a crisp salad. Serves 4-6.

PER SERVING	
calories	409
g fat	7
g protein	8
g carbohydrate	82

Serve as part of a buffet lunch with roast chicken drumsticks, cherry tomatoes or a sliced tomato salad (see page 59), Low-Cal Coleslaw (page 75), Red Pepper, Red Bean and Rice Salad (page 74), and wedges of crisp lettuce. Finish with Spiced Mandarin Gâteau (page 172).

Creamy Curried Potato Salad

Keeping the skin on the potatoes retains valuable vitamins and fibre. Stir in the dressing while the potatoes are still warm so that the dressing is absorbed.

1½ lb	baby new potatoes, scrubbed	675 g
5 fl oz	light crème fraîche	150 ml
¼ tsp	ground coriander	1.25 ml
¼ tsp	ground cumin	1.25 ml
2 tbsp	chopped fresh chives	30 ml
	freshly ground black pepper	

Cook the potatoes in boiling water until tender. Meanwhile, whisk together the crème fraîche and spices in a large bowl. Season to taste.

Drain the potatoes and immediately stir into the dressing. Cover and refrigerate.

Just before serving, stir in the chives. Best eaten the same day. Serves 8.

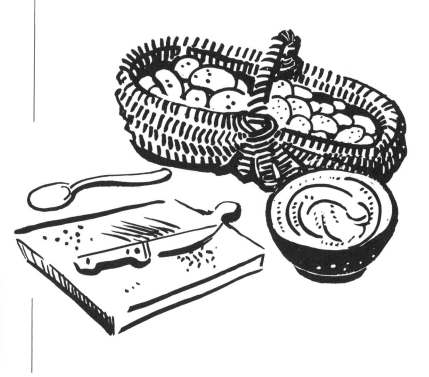

PER SERVING	
calories	78
g fat	2
g protein	2
g carbohydrate	14

As a side dish these spiced vegetables go very well with the Marinated Lamb and Rosemary Kebabs (page 97).

Eastern Spiced Vegetables

I am very fond of vegetable curries and will often choose a vegetarian option when we have an Indian meal. This recipe can also be used as a side dish rather than a main and of course you may vary the low carbohydrate vegetables such as onions, peppers, courgettes, carrots and cauliflower to suit your taste or what you have to hand in the kitchen.

1 tbsp	olive or corn oil	15 ml
1	large onion, sliced	1
1 tbsp	curry powder	15 ml
2 tsp	chilli powder	10 ml
1 tsp	turmeric	5 ml
1	green pepper, deseeded and chopped	1
2	cloves garlic, crushed	2
3	small courgettes, sliced	3
2	large carrots, diced	2
4 oz	baby sweetcorn, sliced	100 g
8 oz	cauliflower, cut into small florets	225 g
1	can (14 oz/400 g) chick peas, drained	1
1	can (14 oz/400 g) tomatoes	1
1/4 pt	water	150 ml
	salt and freshly ground black pepper	

Heat the oil in a large frying pan or wok. Cook the onion, curry powder, chilli and turmeric for 1-2 minutes, stirring constantly. Stir in the remaining ingredients, bring to the boil and simmer, half covered for 20 minutes until the liquid is absorbed. Serve with freshly cooked rice. Serves 4.

PER SERVING	
calories	218
g fat	7
g protein	13
g carbohydrate	27

An enchilada is a tortilla that is rolled around a filling and seasoned with chilli. Enchilada is from the Mexican Spanish enchilado meaning 'seasoned with chilli'.

Chilli Bean Enchiladas

Creating the recipes for this book was the first time I had made tortillas and they were surprisingly easy to make. Tortillas are dry, floury pancakes served with Mexican meals. Each tortilla has 11 g of carbohydrate.

3 oz	plain flour	75 g
2 oz	plain wholemeal flour	50 g
1 tsp	salt	5 ml
1½ oz	soft margarine	40 g
¼ pt	hot water	150 ml
1	can (14 oz/400 g) baked beans	1
1	can (14 oz/400 g) kidney beans, rinsed and drained	1
1-2 tsp	hot chilli powder	5-10 ml
1 tsp	cumin	5 ml
	salt and freshly ground black pepper	
3 oz	cheddar, grated	75 g

Sift the flours together with the salt, tipping any bran remaining in the sieve back into the bowl. Rub in the margarine. Stir in enough water to form a soft but not sticky dough. Knead for 5 minutes until the dough is smooth and elastic. Divide the dough into 8 pieces, shape into balls and flatten slightly. Roll out each piece very thinly on a lightly floured surface to a 6-inch (15-cm) round.

Heat a heavy-based frying pan until a few drops of water sizzle when sprinkled over. Cook the tortillas one at a time for 30-40 seconds, turning over halfway through cooking until they look pale and floury. Wrap the tortillas in a damp teatowel until ready to serve.

Mix together the beans, chilli powder and cumin. Season to taste. Divide the beans among the tortillas and roll up. Place in an ovenproof dish and sprinkle with the cheese. Bake in a preheated oven at 200°C (400°F) Gas Mark 6 for 20 minutes. Serve with a mixed salad. Serves 4.

PER SERVING	
calories	432
g fat	16
g protein	20
g carbohydrate	55

Easy-blend yeast
This quick form of yeast is added to the dry ingredients and must not be soaked in water first. If you have fresh yeast add it to a little of the warm water, add a pinch of flour and a pinch of sugar in a small bowl. Allow to become spongy and then add to the ingredients with the rest of the warm water and oil.

Courgette, Sweetcorn and Red Pepper Pizza

I use a table-top electric mixer to knead the dough, which only takes 1-2 minutes. The dough is enough to make two thin base 9-inch (23-cm) pizzas.

For the base

8 oz	strong plain flour	225 g
1 tsp	easy-blend dried yeast	5 ml
1/4 tsp	salt	1.25 ml
1/4 pt	warm water	150 ml
1 tbsp	olive or sunflower oil	15 ml

For the topping

1 tbsp	olive or sunflower oil	15 ml
1	red onion, sliced	1
2	large courgettes, sliced	2
4 oz	baby sweetcorn, sliced	100 g
2	red peppers, deseeded and diced	2
2	cans (14 oz/400 g) chopped tomatoes, drained	2
1 tbsp	tomato purée	15 ml
2 tbsp	chopped fresh basil	30 ml
6 oz	cheddar, grated	175 g
12	black olives in brine, pitted	12
5-6	fresh basil leaves	5-6

Sift the flour into a large bowl. Stir in the yeast and salt. Make a well in the centre and gradually work in the water and oil to form a soft dough. Knead for 8-10 minutes until smooth and elastic. Place in an oiled bowl, cover and leave to rise in a warm place for 45 minutes until doubled in size.

Meanwhile, heat the oil in a medium-sized saucepan. Add the onion, courgettes, sweetcorn, and peppers and stir-fry for 2-3 minutes. Remove from the heat and set aside. Preheat the oven to 230°C (450°F) Gas Mark 8. Place a large baking sheet on the top shelf of the oven. Knead the risen dough on a lightly floured surface. Roll out into two 9-inch (23-cm) rounds and

PER WHOLE PIZZA	
calories	1038
g fat	50
g protein	44
g carbohydrate	112

press into pizza plates or shallow cake tins.

Mix the drained tomatoes with the tomato purée and chopped basil and spread over the pizza bases, almost to the edge. Top with the cooked vegetables and sprinkle with the cheese, olives and basil leaves.

Place the pizzas on the preheated baking sheet in the oven and cook for 20-25 minutes until the top is bubbling and golden. Serve at once. Makes two 9-inch (23-cm) pizzas.

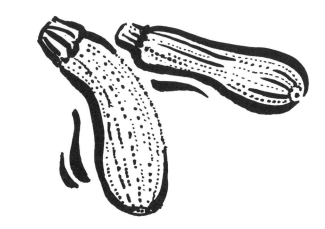

Courgettes Provençales

My mother used to make this dish for our family, and I now use it when entertaining friends. I find the combination of courgettes, onions and tomatoes works well, and it's low in fat and calories too.

2 lb	courgettes, sliced	900 g
2 tsp	olive or sunflower oil	10 ml
1	small onion, finely chopped	1
1	can (14 oz/400 g) chopped tomatoes	1
1 tbsp	tomato purée	15 ml
1 tsp	dried herbes de Provence	5 ml

PER SERVING	
calories	60
g fat	2
g protein	4
g carbohydrate	6

Steam the courgettes over boiling water for 5 minutes, drain. Meanwhile, heat the oil in a small saucepan and cook the onion for 5 minutes until soft. Stir in the drained courgettes, tomatoes, tomato purée and herbs and simmer for 10 minutes. Serve immediately. Serves 6 as an accompaniment.

Mushrooms do not keep well. For them to be at their best use cultivated mushrooms within 2-3 days and use the wild varieties the same day you buy them. Shiitake is wonderful to cook with cultivated mushrooms as the powerful flavour adds to the blander variety.

Three Mushroom Pasta Sauce

Using a mixture of mushrooms gives a variety of size, shape and flavour. Shiitake mushrooms have a distinctive flavour and meaty texture.

1 tbsp	olive or sunflower oil	15 ml
2	cloves garlic, crushed	2
1	medium onion, finely chopped	1
1½ lb	mixed mushrooms such as shiitake chestnut and oyster, sliced	675 g
¼ pt	boiling vegetable stock	150 ml
1 tbsp	cornflour	15 ml
2 tbsp	cold water	30 ml
4 tbsp	dry white wine	60 ml
	salt and freshly ground black pepper	
	chopped fresh parsley to garnish	

Heat the oil in a large non-stick frying pan or wok and cook the garlic, onion and mushrooms for 2-3 minutes, stirring continuously. Add the stock and bring to the boil. Reduce the heat and simmer, uncovered, for 15 minutes, stirring occasionally.

Mix the cornflour and water to a smooth paste and stir into the mushroom mixture with the wine. Season to taste. Boil for 2-3 minutes until the sauce is thickened. Spoon over freshly cooked pasta and garnish with chopped fresh parsley. Serves 3-4.

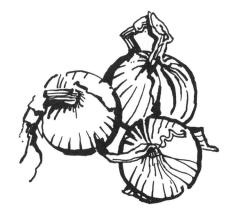

PER SERVING	
calories	112
g fat	6
g protein	4
g carbohydrate	8

This is a great salad for all sorts of buffet parties and barbecues as it can be made and dressed well in advance and will only improve with standing. If you want to add a touch of fresh green at the last minute, sprinkle with a little parsley before serving.

Red Pepper, Red Bean and Rice Salad

I made this for my daughter Jade's Christening buffet and it proved very popular. Using the rice as a base, you can vary the salad vegetables to suit your taste. For example, use spring onions in place of the red onion or tomatoes instead of peppers or cucumber.

6 oz	rice, cooked	175 g
1	small red onion, very finely chopped	1
1	red pepper, finely diced	1
2	sticks celery, sliced	2
1/4	cucumber, diced	1/4
1	can (7½ oz/213 g) kidney beans, rinsed and drained	1
2 oz	sultanas	50 g
1 tbsp	olive oil	15 ml
1 tbsp	white wine vinegar	15 ml
2 tbsp	chopped fresh coriander	30 ml
	salt and freshly ground black pepper	

Mix all the ingredients in a large bowl and season to taste. Turn into a serving bowl and chill until required. Serves 10 as part of a buffet.

PER SERVING	
calories	118
g fat	2
g protein	3
g carbohydrate	23

Low-Fat Waldorf Salad

I use natural yogurt in place of some of the mayonnaise usually used for this dish, to lower the fat content and also the calories. Low-fat natural yogurt has around 1 g of fat and 56 calories per 100 g compared to 28 g of fat and 284 calories in a standard reduced-calorie mayonnaise. And there is 79 g of fat in ordinary mayonnaise! I found it was worth taking the time to compare some of the reduced-calorie mayonnaise now available and found one which had 70% less fat than full-fat mayonnaise.

3	medium red apples	3
2 tbsp	lemon juice	30 ml
2 oz	chopped walnuts	50 g
1	head celery, chopped	1
1	carton (5 oz/150 g) low-fat natural yogurt	1
5 tbsp	reduced-calorie mayonnaise	75 ml

Core the apples and dice, leaving the skins on. Sprinkle with lemon juice to prevent browning. Mix with the walnuts, celery, yogurt and mayonnaise. Mix well to combine. Turn into a serving dish and chill until required. Serves 6.

PER SERVING	
calories	172
g fat	16
g protein	3
g carbohydrate	6

Low-Cal Coleslaw

I always make my own coleslaw as I find the shop bought ones always have an overpowering taste of mayonnaise. I usually serve coleslaw at barbecues and buffets and this amount will make one large bowl which will serve at least 10-12 people. I use a food processor and slicing plate to shred the cabbage which gives a very fine shred and a fine grating plate to grate the carrot which reduces the preparation time considerably.

1	small white cabbage, shredded	1
4	medium carrots, grated	4
6	spring onions, finely chopped	6
10-12 tbsp	reduced-calorie mayonnaise or salad cream	150-180 ml
	a few snipped chives to garnish	

Place all the vegetables into a large bowl. Add the mayonnaise or salad cream and mix well. Turn into a serving bowl and chill before serving. Garnish with a few snipped chives. Serves 10-12.

PER SERVING	
calories	90
g fat	8
g protein	1
g carbohydrate	4

A super midweek supper. This is a very quick dish that you can make for friends on a night after work.

Quick Three Bean Chilli

1 tbsp	olive or sunflower oil	15 ml
1	onion, finely chopped	1
1	clove garlic, crushed	1
1-2 tsp	chilli powder (to taste)	5-10 ml
1 tsp	cumin	5 ml
2 tbsp	tomato purée	30 ml
1	can (14 oz/400 g) chopped tomatoes	1
1	can (14 oz/400 g) butter beans, drained	1
1	can (14 oz/400 g) kidney beans, drained	1
1	can (14 oz/400 g) cannellini beans, drained	1
	salt and freshly ground black pepper	

Heat the oil in a large saucepan, add the onion and garlic and cook for a few minutes. Add the chilli powder, cumin and tomato purée and cook for a few seconds, stirring. Stir in the remaining ingredients, cover and simmer gently for 10-20 minutes or until piping hot. Check the seasoning and serve. Serves 4-6. Serve with rice.

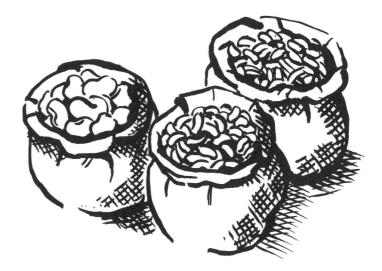

PER SERVING	
calories	312
g fat	5
g protein	20
g carbohydrate	49

Creamy Vegetable Filo Pie

As sheets of filo pastry vary in size between brands, you may need to match the number of sheets to the measurements stated in the recipe. Crumple the pastry over the pie, rather than laying it flat so that you get a crisper result. Brush any remaining fat over the pastry.

1 oz	soft margarine	25 g
1	medium onion, sliced	1
2	courgettes, sliced	2
1	red pepper, deseeded and diced	1
8 oz	broccoli, cut into small florets	225 g
2	large carrots, sliced	2
1 oz	plain flour	25 g
1/2 pt	vegetable stock	275 ml
1/4 pt	semi-skimmed milk	150 ml
1 tsp	dried mixed herbs	5 ml
	salt and freshly ground black pepper	
1	sheet filo pastry 18 x 11 inches (45 x 28 cm)	1
1/2 oz	soft margarine	15 g

Melt the margarine in a large saucepan. Add the onion, courgette, red pepper, broccoli and carrot and cook for 5 minutes, stirring occasionally. Stir in the flour, cook for 1 minute, then gradually add the vegetable stock. Cook for 2 minutes until thickened. Gradually add the milk, herbs and seasoning. Bring to the boil and cook for 2-3 minutes until thickened.

Spoon the mixture into a 2½-pint (1.2-litre) ovenproof dish. Brush one side of the filo pastry with the melted margarine and then tear it into pieces. Arrange the filo pastry over the vegetable mixture with the greased side up. Bake in a preheated oven at 220°C (425°F) Gas Mark 7 for 15 minutes or until golden brown. Serve hot with noodles/new potatoes and salad. Serves 4.

PER SERVING	
calories	174
g fat	10
g protein	6
g carbohydrate	16

Sesame Scones
Make the cobbler topping but bake on a greased baking tray for 20 minutes or until well risen and golden. Serve with grilled meats and a gravy or simply split and buttered for a snack.

Vegetable and Chick Pea Cobbler

A filling main course which is particularly welcome on a cold winter night. Serve with extra vegetables and crusty bread.

For the topping

3 oz	self-raising wholemeal flour	75 g
3 oz	self-raising flour	75 g
	a pinch of salt	
2 oz	soft margarine	50 g
5 tbsp	skimmed milk	75 ml
2 tbsp	sesame seeds	30 ml

For the filling

1 tbsp	olive or sunflower oil	15 ml
1	large onion, peeled and finely diced	1
1	clove garlic, crushed (optional)	1
4	medium carrots, sliced	4
1	small courgette, sliced	1
4 oz	mushrooms, sliced	100 g
2 tsp	mixed dried herbs	10 ml
1/2 tsp	yeast extract	2.5 ml
1 tbsp	tomato purée	15 ml
	salt and freshly ground black pepper	
3/4 pt	water	425 ml
1	can (14 oz/400 g) chick peas	1
1	can (7 oz/200 g) baked beans	1
2 tsp	cornflour	10 ml
2 tbsp	cold water	30 ml
	freshly chopped parsley to garnish	

Sieve the flours and salt into a mixing bowl. (Tip any bran remaining in the sieve into the bowl.) Rub in the margarine until the mixture resembles breadcrumbs. Stir in enough milk to form a soft dough. Roll out on a lightly floured surface to 1/2-inch (1-cm) thick. Cut into 2-inch (5-cm) rounds and sprinkle with the sesame seeds.

Heat the oil in a large saucepan and sauté the onion, garlic (if using), carrot and courgette for 2 minutes. Stir in the mushrooms, herbs, yeast extract, tomato purée, seasoning and water. Bring to the boil and simmer for 5 minutes. Stir in the chick peas and baked beans and cook for a further 5 minutes. Meanwhile, mix the cornflour and water together in a small bowl until blended. Add a little of the hot vegetable liquid and blend together. Add the cornflour mixture to the saucepan and bring to the boil. Cook for a few minutes until the sauce is thickened. Place the vegetable mixture in a large, deep ovenproof dish. Arrange the topping around the outside of the dish. Bake the casserole in a preheated oven at 200°C (400°F) Gas Mark 6 for 30 minutes, or until the topping is golden brown. Serve hot, garnished with chopped parsley. Serves 6.

PER SERVING	
calories	342
g fat	15
g protein	12
g carbohydrate	43

Sweet and Sour Quorn Stir-Fry

Quorn is vegetable in origin, low in fat, and a good source of protein and dietary fibre. It is now produced in cubes or in a minced version. Quorn is available from the chilled cabinets in supermarkets. It requires very little cooking and is particularly suitable for a mid-week stir-fry.

For the sauce		
2 tbsp	cornflour	30 ml
2 tbsp	white wine vinegar	30 ml
2 tbsp	lemon juice	30 ml
3 tbsp	soy sauce	45 ml
2 tbsp	tomato purée	30 ml
9 tbsp	water	135 ml
For the stir-fry		
1 tbsp	olive or corn oil	15 ml
1	packet (9 oz/250 g) Quorn cubes	1
1	green pepper, deseeded and sliced	1
1	red pepper, deseeded and sliced	1
7 oz	beansprouts	200 g

PER SERVING	
calories	202
g fat	8
g protein	13
g carbohydrate	20

Blend the cornflour with the remaining sauce ingredients until smooth. Heat the oil in a wok or non-stick frying pan. Add the quorn and peppers and stir fry for 3-4 minutes. Reduce the heat and pour in the sauce. Stir continuously for a few minutes until the sauce is thickened. Stir in the beansprouts and cook for a further 3-4 minutes. Serve with freshly cooked rice or noodles. Serves 3.

Festive Pine Nut Roast

This makes a delicious vegetarian option for Christmas dinner or other special occasion served with potatoes and freshly cooked vegetables and a tomato sauce with basil (see next recipe).

1 tbsp	olive or sunflower oil	15 ml
1	medium onion, finely chopped	1
4 oz	pinenuts	100 g
2 oz	cashew nuts, roughly chopped	50 g
2 oz	Cheshire cheese, grated	50 g
4 oz	fresh wholemeal breadcrumbs	100 g
1 tbsp	fresh chopped parsley or 1 tsp (5 ml) mixed dried herbs	15 ml
2	eggs, beaten	2
	a pinch of ground nutmeg	
	salt and freshly ground black pepper	
For the filling		
1	large carrot, peeled and finely diced	1
1	courgette, finely diced	1
1	small red pepper, deseeded and finely diced	1
To garnish		
	lemon slices and parsley	

Heat the oil in a saucepan, add the onion and gently cook for 5 minutes until soft and golden brown. Remove from the heat, drain and turn into a large bowl. Add the nuts, grated cheese, breadcrumbs, parsley, eggs and seasoning to the onion and mix thoroughly. Quickly stir fry the vegetables for the filling in the remaining oil until just soft. Place half the nut mixture into a lightly greased and base-lined 2 lb (900 g) loaf tin. Cover with the stir-fry vegetables, pressing down well. Top with the remaining nut mixture, press down well and smooth the surface. Bake in a preheated oven at 180°C (350°F) Gas Mark 4 for 45-60 minutes. Remove from the oven and leave to stand in the tin for 5 minutes. Turn out carefully on to a serving dish. Garnish with lemon slices and parsley. Serve with fresh vegetables and potatoes, accompanied by tomato sauce with basil if desired. Serves 6.

Tomato Sauce with Basil

This fat-free sauce is to accompany the Festive Pine Nut Roast, (page 80) but you could also use it as a sauce for pasta.

1	can (14 oz/400 g) chopped tomatoes	1
1-2	cloves garlic, crushed	1-2
2 tbsp	red wine (optional)	30 ml
2 tbsp	fresh basil, chopped	30 ml
	salt and freshly ground black pepper	

Place all the ingredients in a saucepan. Bring to the boil and simmer, uncovered for about 10 minutes until thick, stirring occasionally. Check seasoning and serve hot with the Festive Pine Nut Roast. Serves 6.

PER SERVING	
calories	272
g fat	24
g protein	10
g carbohydrate	6

Suitable for freezing. Make this sauce in the summer when fresh basil is growing well and freeze it for Christmas.

PER SERVING	
calories	14
g fat	1
g protein	1
g carbohydrate	2

Vegetarian Supper Party for 6
*Spinach and Lentil Roulade
(page 82) served with crusty
bread, grilled flat mushrooms
and a green salad.
Tropical Paradise Fruit Salad
(page 205)*

Spinach and Lentil Roulade

This colourful dish makes a very attractive centrepiece to the
table when entertaining. It is also very nutritious and is rich in
vitamin A and potassium.

3 oz	red lentils	75 g
1	small onion, chopped	1
1 tbsp	tomato purée	15 ml
1/2 tsp	cumin (optional)	2.5 ml
1 lb	frozen spinach, defrosted	450 g
1 oz	soft margarine	25 g
1 oz	flour	25 g
1/2 pt	skimmed milk	275 ml
2	eggs, separated	2

Grease and line an 11-inch (28-cm) Swiss roll tin. Bring the
lentils to the boil in plenty of unsalted water. Boil fast for 10
minutes, then rinse and drain. Return to the pan, add the onion
and cook uncovered until tender. Continue heating to evaporate
any excess moisture. Add the tomato purée and cumin (if using),
and season to taste.

Cook the spinach in a saucepan without any added water for
3-4 minutes. Turn into a colander or sieve and press well to
remove as much liquid as possible. Make the white sauce: place
the margarine, flour and milk in a saucepan. Whisk continuously
over a gentle heat until the sauce thickens.

Stir in the spinach and egg yolks and season to taste. Whisk
the egg whites and gently fold into the spinach mixture. Spoon
into the prepared tin and level the top. Bake for 20-25 minutes
at 200°C (400°F) Gas Mark 6 or until golden brown. Turn out on
to non-stick baking parchment. Spread the lentil purée over the
surface and roll up like a Swiss roll. Return to the oven for 5-10
minutes. Serve hot with couscous, potatoes and rice. Serves 4.

PER SERVING	
calories	228
g fat	10
g protein	14
g carbohydrate	20

Suitable for freezing.
*Freeze before baking. Thaw
completely and then bake as in
the recipe.*

Mushroom and Spinach Lasagne

Vegetable lasagne is very easy to make and can be varied to suit your taste or what is available fresh in season. Alternatively, if you wish to use beans to make the dish more filling and increase the fibre content, the lasagne can be served with crusty bread.

For the filling

1 tbsp	olive or sunflower oil	15 ml
1	onion, sliced	1
1	clove garlic, crushed	1
2	medium carrots, thinly sliced	2
4 oz	button mushrooms, sliced	100 g
1	can (14 oz/400 g) tomatoes	1
1 tsp	dried mixed herbs	5 ml
	salt and freshly ground black pepper	
8 oz	frozen chopped spinach, defrosted and drained	225 g
6-8	sheets 'no-pre-cook' lasagne	6-8

For the sauce

1/2 oz	soft margarine	15 g
1/2 oz	plain flour	15 g
1/4 pt	skimmed milk	150 ml
1 oz	cheddar, grated	25 g

For the topping

1 oz	cheddar, grated	25 g
1 oz	unsalted cashew nuts	25 g

Heat the oil in a large saucepan and cook the onion and garlic over a moderate heat for a few minutes. Add the carrot and mushrooms and cook for 5 minutes, stirring frequently. Stir in the tomatoes, herbs and season to taste. Simmer for 5-10 minutes, stirring occasionally.

Meanwhile, make the sauce. Melt the margarine in a small saucepan. Stir in the flour and cook for 1 minute. Gradually stir in the milk and bring to the boil, stirring continuously until thickened. Stir in the cheese and season to taste.

Arrange the vegetable mixture, spinach and lasagne in alternate layers in an oblong dish, ending with a layer of lasagne. Cover with the cheese sauce and scatter the grated cheese and cashew nuts over the top.

Cook in a preheated oven at 180°C (350°F) Gas Mark 4 for 30-35 minutes until golden brown. Serves 4.

PER SERVING	
calories	307
g fat	15
g protein	12
g carbohydrate	32

Couscous and Apricot Salad

Couscous is coarsely ground wheat that is much used in North African cooking. It is semolina from hard durum wheat where the grains have been rolled, dampened and coated with a finer flour to keep them separate during cooking. It has a delicious nutty flavour, is tender and yet retains firm separate grains in texture.

If you do not have a steamer, simply place the couscous in a metal colander and steam over a pan of boiling water. Couscous is available from supermarkets or health food stores and has a carbohydrate value of around 2 oz (50 g) per 4 oz (100 g) weight.

8 oz	couscous	225 g
14 fl oz	boiling water	400 ml
1/2 tsp	salt	2.5 ml
1 tbsp	olive or corn oil	15 ml
1	red pepper, deseeded and finely diced	1
3 oz	dried, ready-to-eat apricots, finely chopped	75 g
2 oz	currants	50 g
1 oz	flaked almonds	25 g
2 tbsp	chopped fresh coriander	30 ml
	salt and freshly ground black pepper	

Place the couscous in a bowl and pour over the water, salt and oil. Cover and allow to stand for 5 minutes. Transfer to a steamer and steam for 6-7 minutes. Separate the grains and turn into a large bowl. Add the remaining ingredients and toss together lightly to mix. Season to taste. Turn into a serving bowl and chill before serving. Serves 6.

PER SERVING	
calories	225
g fat	6
g protein	4
g carbohydrate	40

Pasta with Courgette, Red Pepper and Sweetcorn Sauce

A quick and simple dish which can easily be prepared on returning home from work. Use a vegetarian cheddar cheese in place of the Edam if you prefer. Serve with freshly cooked pasta; a serving of 2 oz (50 g) dried weight gives approximately 35 g carbohydrate.

1 tbsp	olive or corn oil	15 ml
1	onion, sliced	1
1	clove garlic, crushed	1
2	small courgettes, sliced	2
1	red pepper, deseeded and chopped	1
4 oz	baby sweetcorn, sliced	100 g
1 tsp	dried basil	5 ml
1	14 oz (400 g) can chopped tomatoes	1
4 oz	pasta shapes	100 g
	salt and freshly ground black pepper	
2 oz	grated Edam cheese	50 g

Heat the oil in a large non-stick frying pan or wok and cook the onion and garlic for 5 minutes until soft. Add the courgette, pepper, sweetcorn and basil and cook for a further 3-4 minutes. Drain off about 4 tbsp (60 ml) of juice from the tomatoes. Add the tomatoes to the vegetables, season to taste and bring to the boil. Cook, half covered over a moderate heat for 10 minutes until the sauce thickens and the vegetables are just cooked.

Meanwhile, cook the pasta according to the pack instructions. Drain. Toss through the sauce and place in individual serving bowls. Sprinkle the grated cheese over the top. Serve with a fresh crisp salad. Serves 2.

PER SERVING	
calories	421
g fat	16
g protein	19
g carbohydrate	55

This dish captures all the sunshine of Provence in the traditional Provençal ingredients of tomatoes, peppers, aubergines, olive oil and courgettes. If you wish for a really authentic flavour add 1-2 cloves of crushed garlic with the onion and use 2 teaspoons of fresh chopped basil.

Pasta Provençale

I was always taught to salt aubergines before using them in a recipe to remove the bitter juices. However, the Fresh Fruit and Vegetable Information Bureau told me that you don't need to do this anymore with the varieties which are available in the UK.

1 tbsp	olive or sunflower oil	15 ml
1	medium aubergine, chopped	1
1	medium red pepper, deseeded and diced	1
2	medium courgettes, sliced	2
1	large onion, finely chopped	1
1	can (14 oz/400 g) chopped tomatoes	1
1/4 pt	hot vegetable stock	150 ml
1 tbsp	tomato purée	15 ml
1/2 tsp	dried oregano	2.5 ml
1/2 tsp	dried basil	2.5 ml
	salt and freshly ground black pepper	
9 oz	pasta shapes	250 g

Heat the oil in a medium-sized saucepan, add the aubergine, pepper, courgette, and onion and cook for 5 minutes until soft, stirring occasionally. Add the tomatoes, stock, purée and herbs and season to taste. Cover and simmer for 30 minutes.

Cook the pasta in boiling salted water for 10-15 minutes or according to the packet instructions, until tender, yet firm. Drain. Toss into the Provençale mixture and serve immediately. Serve with a salad. Serves 4.

PER SERVING	
calories	303
g fat	6
g protein	11
g carbohydrate	56

Meat

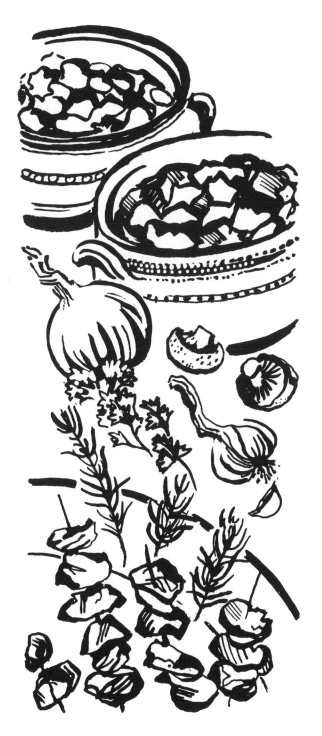

I've tried to use different meats, ranging from liver to game and have also included a lot of poultry recipes. The emphasis is on Mediterranean flavours and includes dishes such as Greek lamb kebabs, and Pastitsio but there are some traditional hearty hotpots and casseroles with beer or dumplings too.

Winter Supper for 4
*Beef casserole with Herby
Dumplings (page 88) served
with jacket potatoes and
steamed wedges of cabbage or
Brussels sprouts
Pears with Raspberry Sauce
(page 165)*

Beef Casserole with Herby Dumplings

This recipe enables the fat content to be cut down by placing all the ingredients in the casserole dish rather than frying the meat first. The long, slow cooking means that the meat is still tender.

1 lb	lean braising steak, fat removed and cubed	450 g
8 oz	swede, peeled and diced	225 g
8 oz	baby onions or shallots, peeled	225 g
5 oz	button mushrooms, halved	150 g
2	large carrots, sliced	2
1	bouquet garni	1
1 pt	boiling beef stock	550 ml
1 tbsp	Worcestershire sauce	15 ml
For the dumplings		
3 oz	self-raising flour	75 g
1 oz	shredded suet	25 g
2 tsp	dried mixed herbs	10 ml
	salt and freshly ground black pepper	

Place the braising steak, vegetables, bouquet garni, stock and Worcestershire sauce in a large ovenproof casserole dish. Season to taste. Bring to the boil on the hob. Cover and transfer to a preheated oven at 180°C (350°F) Gas Mark 4 for 1 hour, stirring occasionally.

Mix together all the ingredients for the dumplings in a small bowl. Add enough water to form a soft elastic dough. With floured hands, form 8 balls. Add to the casserole after 1 hour of cooking. Cook for a further 1 hour stirring occasionally. Remove the bouquet garni before serving. Serve with a jacket potato and freshly cooked vegetables. Serves 4.

PER SERVING	
calories	298
g fat	12
g protein	27
g carbohydrate	22

The word hotpot has had a chequered history. Originally it was a boiled mixture of ale and spirits, usually brandy but by the middle of the 19th century it had become a traditional Lancashire dish of meat and vegetables topped with potatoes. It is most usually lamb that is used but any meat available has been included over the years. For a change try using lean pork and adding a few apple slices under the potato.

Lamb and Lentil Hotpot

Using pulses such as lentils adds extra fibre to casserole dishes and also helps to 'expand' the dish so that less meat is required. Lentils are low in fat and a good source of protein. Unlike most dried pulses, they do not require soaking overnight before use.

2 tbsp	plain flour	30 ml
	salt and freshly ground black pepper	
2 tsp	dried rosemary	10 ml
1¼ lb	lean braising lamb, fat removed, cut into cubes	550 g
4 oz	red lentils	100 g
1	large onion, finely diced	1
8 oz	carrots, sliced	225 g
12 oz	swede, diced	350 g
1¼ pt	boiling beef stock	700 ml
1½ lb	potatoes	675 g
1 tbsp	olive or corn oil	15 ml

Season the flour with the salt and pepper and rosemary. Toss the lamb in the flour to coat evenly. Place in an ovenproof casserole dish.

Boil the lentils fast in boiling water for 10 minutes. Drain, rinse and drain again. Add to the casserole dish with the onion, carrot, swede and stock. Mix well. Bring to the boil on the hob. cover and transfer to a preheated oven at 160°C (325°F) Gas Mark 3 for 1½ hours. Peel the potatoes and thinly slice. Arrange on top of the casserole to cover the top and brush with the oil.

Return to the oven and cook uncovered for 1 hour. Serve hot with freshly cooked vegetables. Serves 4.

PER SERVING	
calories	579
g fat	16
g protein	52
g carbohydrate	60

Lambs' liver is one of the best buys in offal. It is full of flavour but not strong and coarse. While not quite as tender and delicate as calves' liver it is not nearly as expensive. It is one of the very best sources of iron as the type of iron it contains is used by the body most efficiently.

Lambs' Liver with Spicy Tomato Sauce

A simple and economical meal. Serve with potatoes and freshly cooked vegetables.

1¼ lb	lambs' liver, sliced	550 g
1 tbsp	seasoned flour	15 ml
2 tbsp	olive or sunflower oil	30 ml
1	large onion	1
3	sticks celery, finely sliced	3
½ tsp	paprika	2.5 ml
1	can (14 oz/400 g) chopped tomatoes	1

Dust the liver with the flour. Heat the oil in a non-stick frying pan, and cook the liver, turning until the liver has changed colour. Add the onion and celery and cook over a gentle heat. Stir in the remaining ingredients. Cover and simmer for approximately 10-15 minutes. Serve hot. Serves 4.

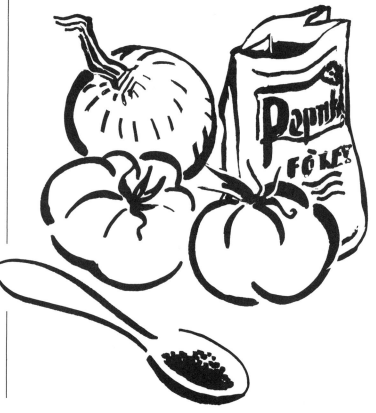

PER SERVING	
calories	370
g fat	22
g protein	30
g carbohydrate	14

Right:
Lamb and Lentil Hotpot
(page 89)

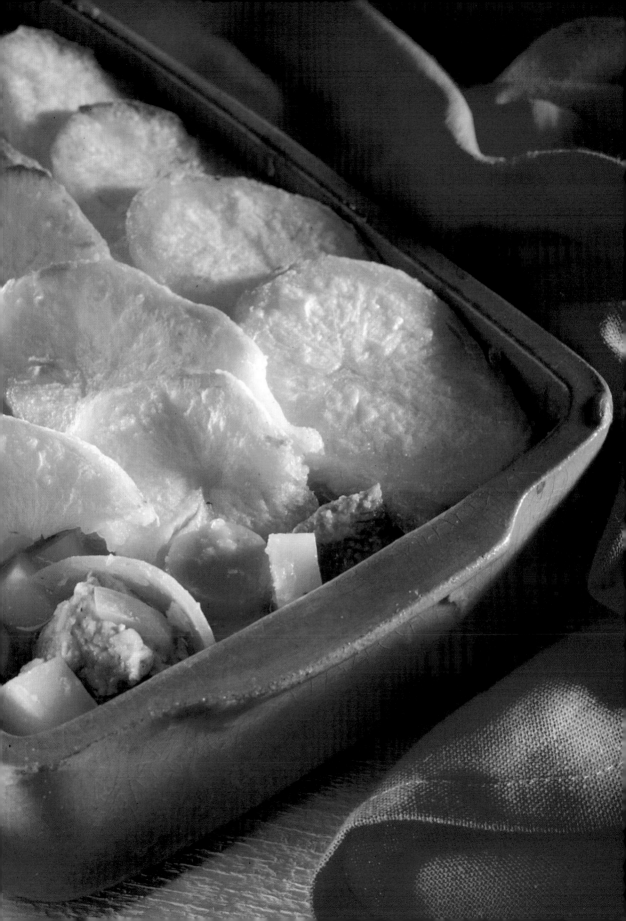

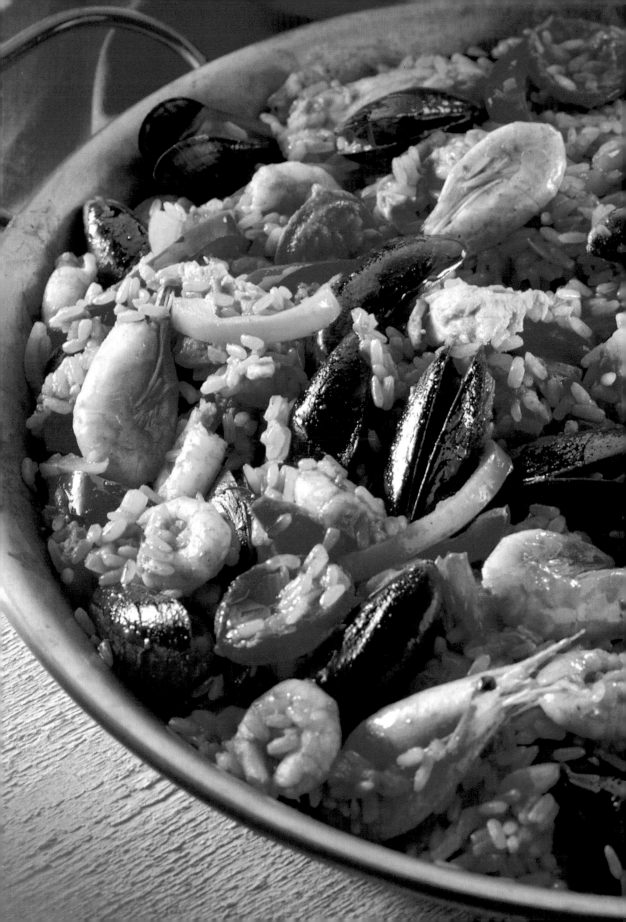

Creamy Leek and Ham Tart

A delicious creamy tart which may be eaten hot or cold.

For the pastry

4 oz	plain wholemeal flour	100 g
4 oz	plain flour	100 g
	a pinch of salt	
2 oz	polyunsaturated white vegetable fat (such as Flora)	50 g
2 oz	soft margarine	50 g

For the filling

8 oz	leeks, thinly sliced	225 g
3/4 pt	skimmed milk	425 ml
1 oz	plain flour	25 g
1 oz	soft margarine	25 g
2 oz	cheddar, grated	50 g
2	eggs, beaten	2
2 oz	lean ham, chopped	50 g
	freshly ground black pepper	

Sift the flours and salt into a bowl, (tip any bran remaining in the sieve into the bowl). Rub in the pastry fats until the mixture resembles breadcrumbs. Add enough water to mix to a soft dough, about 3 tbsp (45 ml). Roll out on a lightly floured surface to line a deep 9-inch (23-cm) flan ring. Chill for 10 minutes. Prick the base and bake blind at 200°C (400°F) Gas Mark 6 for 10 minutes. Remove the baking beans and greaseproof paper and cook for a further 5 minutes. Reduce the heat to 190°C (375°F) Gas Mark 5.

Cook the leeks in boiling water for 10 minutes. Drain and set aside.

Place the milk, flour and soft margarine in a saucepan and cook over a gentle heat, whisking continuously. Bring to the boil and continue cooking for 1-2 minutes until thick. Remove from the heat and add the cheese and eggs. Whisk together until smooth. Season well. Fold in the leeks and ham. Spoon into the cooked flan case. Bake in the preheated oven for 35-40 minutes until golden. Serves 8.

PER SERVING	
calories	287
g fat	18
g protein	10
g carbohydrate	24

Left:
Chicken, Spicy Sausage and Seafood Paella (page 103)

Pilau or Pilaf, as it is sometimes called, is usually made with rice. This variation made with couscous (see page 84) is a perfect foil for the Moorish flavours of the chicken brochettes.

Spiced Chicken Brochettes with Couscous, Red Bean and Coriander Pilau

A brochette is simply the name for a skewer on which chunks of meat are cooked. The chicken benefits from being marinated for at least 2 hours or overnight so that all the lovely flavours can develop.

4	5 oz (150 g) boneless, skinless chicken breasts	4
6 tbsp	lemon juice	90 ml
2 tbsp	olive oil	30 ml
1 tsp	paprika	5 ml
	freshly ground black pepper	
1 tsp	ground cumin	5 ml
2 tsp	ground coriander	10 ml
8 oz	couscous	225 g
7 fl oz	cold water	200 ml
1/2 tsp	salt	2.5 ml
1	can (7 oz/200 g) red kidney beans, drained and rinsed	1
1 oz	sultanas	25 g
4 tbsp	fresh coriander, chopped	60 ml
	lemon wedges to garnish	

Soak 8 wooden skewers in hot water for 3 minutes to prevent burning during cooking. Slice the chicken breasts in half lengthways and thread one strip of chicken on to each wooden skewer. Place in a shallow dish. Mix together the lemon juice, 1 tbsp (15 ml) of the olive oil, the paprika, pepper, cumin and coriander in a small bowl. Spoon over the chicken and marinate in the refrigerator for 2 hours.

Place the couscous in a large bowl and stir in the water and salt. Leave to soak for 5 minutes, then add another 7 fl oz (200 ml) water and the remaining olive oil.

Stir well with a fork to break up any lumps. Leave to stand for a further 10 minutes, or until the grains are slightly swollen.

Place the chicken breasts under a hot grill and grill for 15-20 minutes, turning occasionally. Brush with the marinade during cooking.

PER SERVING	
calories	524
g fat	15
g protein	40
g carbohydrate	62

Meanwhile, put the couscous in a fine metal sieve or colander and steam for 10 minutes. Stir in the kidney beans and sultanas and steam for a further 5 minutes. Stir in half the coriander and spoon into a serving dish. Arrange the chicken brochettes over the top and serve garnished with the remaining coriander and lemon wedges. Serves 4.

Low-Fat Pastitsio

Pasta is most usually thought of as an Italian dish but before the fourth century when Latin cookery books record the word to mean dough, it was a food used by the Greeks and their word meant 'barley porridge'. Macaroni has been around since the sixteenth century. Macaroni is, in fact, a Greek word meaning 'food made from barley'. This Greek pasta dish is, therefore, very much an ancient speciality.

This is a spicy Greek dish which I have adapted to lower the fat content without affecting the flavour. Serve with a fresh green salad.

1 lb	lean minced lamb	450 g
1	large onion, finely chopped	1
2	garlic cloves, crushed	2
1 tsp	dried oregano	5 ml
1 tsp	dried thyme	5 ml
1/2 tsp	ground cinnamon	2.5 ml
1 tsp	ground cumin	5 ml
	a pinch of ground ginger	
	a pinch of grated nutmeg	
1	bay leaf	1
1/4 pt	dry white wine	150 ml
1	can (14 oz/400 g) chopped tomatoes	1
1 tbsp	tomato purée	15 ml
	salt and freshly ground black pepper	
6 oz	pasta	175 g
2 tbsp	freshly chopped coriander (optional)	30 ml
1 oz	soft margarine	25 g
1 oz	plain flour	25 g
12 fl oz	skimmed milk	350 ml
2 oz	cheddar, grated	50 g
1	egg, beaten	1

Place the lamb in a large non-stick pan with the onion and garlic and cook over a moderate heat for 5 minutes until browned. Stir in the herbs, spices and bay leaf, and cook for a further 5 minutes, stirring occasionally.

Stir in the wine, tomatoes, tomato purée and seasoning. Bring to the boil, half cover and simmer for 30 minutes, stirring occasionally, until the sauce is thickened and well reduced. Season to taste.

Meanwhile, cook the pasta in boiling, salted water until just tender. Drain and stir into the lamb mixture with the chopped coriander, if using. Spoon into a large shallow 2-pt (1-litre) ovenproof dish.

Place the margarine in a saucepan with the flour and milk. Whisk continuously over a moderate heat until thickened. Remove from the heat and allow to cool slightly. Beat in the cheese and egg. Season to taste. Pour over the lamb mixture. Cook in a preheated oven at 190°C (375°F) Gas Mark 5 for 35-40 minutes or until golden brown and piping hot. Serve hot with a green salad, and crusty bread if desired. Serves 4-6.

PER SERVING	
calories	571
g fat	22
g protein	40
g carbohydrate	52

Beef, Pepper and Baby Sweetcorn Stir-Fry

This recipe is ideal for entertaining as most of the preparation can be done in advance leaving you more time with your guests. I marinate the meat in the morning and prepare the vegetables just before our guests arrive.

1 lb	lean fillet steak, sliced into very thin strips	450 g
1 tbsp	cornflour	15 ml
2 tbsp	soy sauce	30 ml
6 tbsp	dry red wine	90 ml
3 tbsp	red wine vinegar	45 ml
	salt and freshly ground black pepper	
1 tbsp	olive or corn oil	15 ml
1	onion, finely sliced	1
2	cloves garlic, crushed	2
1-inch	piece fresh root ginger, grated	2.5-cm
3	sticks celery, finely sliced	3

Fillet steak is expensive but for this recipe, where it is to be cut into strips, see if you can buy a tail end piece of fillet. It should be cheaper than the thick end.

Oriental Supper for 4
Cheese and Spinach Filo Triangles (page 35)
Beef, Pepper and Baby Sweetcorn Stir-Fry (page 94) served with noodles or rice
Figs with Blackberry Sauce (page 170)

1	red pepper, deseeded and finely sliced	1
1	green pepper, deseeded and finely sliced	1
8 oz	baby sweetcorn, cut into small pieces	225 g
4 oz	chestnut mushrooms, sliced	100 g

Place the steak in a bowl. Mix together the cornflour, soy sauce, wine and vinegar and season to taste. Pour over the meat, stir well to coat, cover and leave to marinate for 2 hours or overnight.

Heat the oil in a wok or large frying pan. Add the onion, garlic and ginger and stir-fry over a moderate heat for 2-3 minutes. Drain the marinade from the steak and reserve, add the meat to the wok and stir-fry over a high heat for 3-4 minutes. Add the remaining vegetables and stir fry for 2-3 minutes.

Add the marinade and stir until bubbling and well mixed. Adjust seasoning to taste and serve immediately. Serve with freshly cooked noodles or rice. Serves 4.

PER SERVING	
calories	296
g fat	11
g protein	36
g carbohydrate	8

30-minute Supper

Quick Chick Pea Dip served with vegetable crudités (page 24)
Thirty-Minute Meatballs (page 95) served with pasta
Peach Crunch (page 182)

Thirty-Minute Meatballs

If you can't find fresh oregano in the shops, use 2 teaspoons of dried oregano instead. Chop the onion very finely or the mixture will be more difficult to form into balls.

1 lb	extra-lean minced beef	450 g
1	onion, very finely chopped	1
2 tbsp	freshly chopped oregano	30 ml
	salt and freshly ground black pepper	
2	cloves garlic, crushed	2
1/2 pt	Passata (see page 121)	275 ml
1/4 pt	dry red wine	150 ml
1	red pepper, deseeded and finely chopped	1
1	green pepper, deseeded and finely chopped	1

Mix the mince, onion, oregano and seasoning together in a large bowl. Using wet hands, shape the mixture into approximately 16 balls. Chill in the refrigerator until required.

Place the remaining ingredients in a large saucepan and simmer gently for 5 minutes. Add seasoning to taste. Add the meatballs, bring to the boil, cover and simmer for 20 minutes until cooked. Serve with freshly cooked pasta. Serves 4.

PER SERVING	
calories	232
g fat	12
g protein	16
g carbohydrate	9

Chuck or blade steak are the best of the meats for stewing and casseroling. They are also good for braising and often sold labelled as braising steak. For a cheaper alternative, that does add to the rich quality of a long-cooked casserole, look for shin of beef.

Rich Beef Casserole with Stout

A rich tasting casserole which is perfect for winter evenings. The stout can be replaced with stock if preferred.

1 tbsp	olive or sunflower oil	15 ml
2 lb	lean braising steak, trimmed and cubed	900 g
2	cloves garlic, crushed	2
2	large onions, sliced	2
2	large carrots, peeled and sliced	2
8 oz	button mushrooms, halved	225 g
1 tbsp	plain flour	15 ml
3/4 pt	boiling beef stock	425 ml
1/4 pt	stout	150 ml
1	bay leaf	1
1 tsp	dried mixed herbs	5 ml
	salt and freshly ground black pepper	

Heat the oil in a large flameproof casserole dish and cook the meat, garlic and onion for 10 minutes until the meat is browned. Add the carrot and mushrooms and cook for 5 minutes until softened. Add the flour and stir well. Pour in the hot stock and stout and stir well. Add the bay leaf and herbs and season to taste. Bring to the boil, cover and transfer to a preheated oven at 180°C (350°F) Gas Mark 4. Cook for 2 1/2 hours until the meat is tender. Stir occasionally during cooking. Serve with jacket potatoes and freshly cooked vegetables. Serves 4-6.

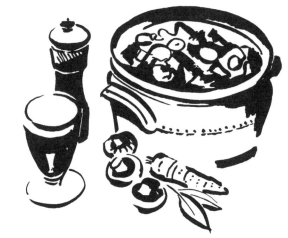

PER SERVING	
calories	492
g fat	18
g protein	67
g carbohydrate	15

Marinated Lamb and Rosemary Kebabs

This simple dish is ideal for barbecues. Serve with a Greek salad (see page 58) and freshly cooked rice or couscous.

1½ lb	lean lamb shoulder steaks, trimmed and cubed	675 g
3 tbsp	olive oil	45 ml
3 tbsp	lemon juice	45 ml
2 tbsp	fresh rosemary	30 ml
	freshly ground black pepper	

Thread the meat on to metal skewers and lay in a shallow dish. Mix the oil, lemon juice, rosemary and pepper together and pour the marinade over the kebabs. Chill for 2 hours. Grill the kebabs under a hot grill for approximately 10-15 minutes, brushing with the marinade and turning frequently. Serve hot. Serves 4.

PER SERVING	
calories	386
g fat	25
g protein	39
g carbohydrate	0

Boeuf Bourguignon

A classic Burgundy dish. The flavour improves if it is made a day in advance and kept in the refrigerator.

2 tbsp	olive oil	30 ml
2 lb	lean braising steak, cubed	900 g
4 oz	lean back bacon, chopped	100 g
3	sticks celery, sliced	3
4	carrots, sliced	4
2	cloves garlic, crushed	2
1 tbsp	plain flour	15 ml
1 pt	beef stock	550 ml
¼ pt	dry red wine	150 ml
1	bay leaf	1
1	bouquet garni	1
	salt and freshly ground black pepper	

Heat the oil in a large pan and cook the meat a few pieces at a time until browned. Drain and transfer to a large casserole dish. Cook the bacon, celery, carrot and garlic in the remaining oil for 2 minutes.

Stir the flour into the pan and cook for 1 minute, stirring constantly. Gradually add the stock, wine, bay leaf, bouquet garni and seasoning. Bring to the boil and pour over the meat. cover and cook in a preheated oven at 180°C (350°F) Gas Mark 4 for 2½ hours. Stir in the onions 30 minutes before the end of cooking time. Remove the bouquet garni and bay leaf and adjust seasoning if necessary. Serve with boiled potatoes in their skins, fresh vegetables and crusty bread if desired. Serves 5.

PER SERVING	
calories	426
g fat	18
g protein	56
g carbohydrate	10

Suitable for freezing.
Use within 3 months. Defrost thoroughly before reheating until piping hot right through.

Chicken Burgundy

A traditional French coq au vin. Don't be put off by the large amount of wine used as most of the alcohol evaporates during cooking.

2 tbsp	olive oil	30 ml
4	boneless chicken breasts, skin removed	4
12	baby onions, sliced	12
2	cloves garlic, crushed	2
4	rashers, lean back bacon, chopped	4
5 oz	button mushrooms, halved	150 g
1 tbsp	plain flour	15 ml
³/₄ pt	boiling chicken stock	425 ml
½ pt	dry red burgundy wine	275 ml
1	bouquet garni	1
	salt and freshly ground black pepper	
2 tbsp	chopped fresh parsley	30 ml

Heat the oil in a large pan and cook the chicken pieces until browned, turning occasionally. Drain and transfer the chicken to a large casserole dish with lid.

Cook the onion, garlic and bacon in the remaining oil until golden. Spoon into the casserole dish. Cook the mushrooms for 2-3 minutes. Add the flour and cook for 1 minute stirring. Gradually add the chicken stock, wine, bouquet garni, and seasoning. Bring to the boil, then pour over the chicken pieces. Cover and cook in a preheated oven at 180°C (350°F) Gas Mark 4 for 1 hour or until the chicken is tender. Remove the bouquet garni and sprinkle with chopped parsley. Serve with crusty bread or boiled potatoes and fresh vegetables. Serves 4.

PER SERVING	
calories	294
g fat	13
g protein	25
g carbohydrate	6

Fast Food for 2
So often fast food seems to mean convenience packets or takeaways. Here is a jiffy meal for a couple in just a couple of ticks. You could prepare and cook this one evening quicker than you could drive to the local takeaway and it is vibrant with natural colour and vitamins not artificial additives. Make up the quantity of Salsa and keep it in the fridge for dipping during the week.

Quick Tomato Salsa (page 26) served with tortilla chips
Shredded Gammon and Pineapple Stir-Fry (page 99) served with pasta
Figs with Blackberry Sauce – half the recipe (page 170)

Shredded Gammon and Pineapple Stir-Fry

A colourful stir-fry which also tastes delicious. Use canned pineapple in natural juice rather than in syrup to cut down on the sugar content.

1 tbsp	olive or sunflower oil	15 ml
6 oz	lean gammon steak, trimmed and cut into thin strips	175 g
½	red pepper, deseeded and sliced	½
½	green pepper, deseeded and sliced	½
4 oz	baby sweetcorn, sliced	100 g
	freshly ground black pepper	
1	can (8 oz/225 g) pineapple pieces in natural juice, drained and juice reserved	1
2 tsp	cornflour	10 ml

Heat the oil in a frying pan or wok, add the gammon and cook for 1-2 minutes until slightly browned. Add the peppers, sweetcorn and seasoning and cook for 2-3 minutes. Mix the cornflour with a little of the reserved pineapple juice and add to the stir-fry with remaining juice and pineapple. Cook over a high heat for a few minutes until the sauce has thickened. Serve immediately with freshly cooked pasta. Serves 2.

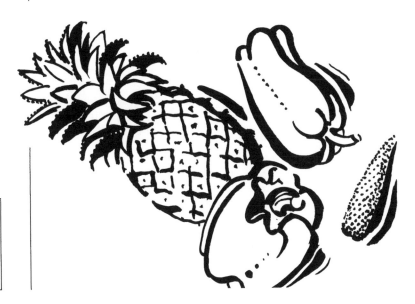

PER SERVING	
calories	294
g fat	12
g protein	30
g carbohydrate	16

Pinto beans are an important ingredient in Mexican cooking. They are an attractive variation of a kidney bean. They have a pale pink skin and small brown blotches or speckles. This has led to their name 'pinto' which, in Mexican Spanish means 'painted'.

Lamb and Apricot Casserole

This recipe includes pinto beans and dried apricots to replace some of the meat. This has several advantages including lowering the cost, reducing the fat content and increasing the amount of fibre. They also add a richness to the sauce and make the meal more filling.

1 tbsp	olive or corn oil	15 ml
1 lb	lean fillet of lamb, cubed	450 g
1	large onion, finely chopped	1
1	medium green pepper, deseeded and sliced	1
1	medium red pepper, deseeded and sliced	1
1 tbsp	plain flour	15 ml
1	can (14 oz/400 g) pinto beans, drained	1
1 tsp	turmeric	5 ml
	salt and freshly ground black pepper	
1 pt	boiling meat stock	550 ml
3 oz	dried ready-to-eat apricots, chopped	75 g
1 tbsp	lemon juice	15 ml

Heat the oil in a flameproof casserole over a moderate heat. Add the lamb and onion and cook for 5 minutes until the lamb is browned, stirring constantly. Add the peppers and cook for a further 2 minutes. Stir in the flour, beans, turmeric and seasoning. Gradually stir in the stock. Bring to the boil, cover and transfer to a preheated oven at 180°C (350°F) Gas Mark 4 for 1 hour. Stir in the apricots and lemon juice. Add a little more stock if becoming too dry. Return to the oven for a further 15 minutes. Serve immediately with potatoes and freshly cooked vegetables. Serves 4.

PER SERVING	
calories	385
g fat	14
g protein	32
g carbohydrate	33

Cajun seasoning is a hot spicy mixture redolent of the American Deep South. It is basically a seasoned salt so you won't need to add any more salt to the dish but it also contains a powerful blend of herbs and spices. These include chilli powder and dried pimentos, pepper, garlic, allspice, coriander seed, cumin, fennel seed, cardamom, mustard, thyme, sage and oregano.

Georgia Chicken

The peanuts add an unexpected bite to the sauce and make it a little bit different. Cajun seasoning is available from supermarkets in the spice section.

4	medium chicken breast fillets, skin removed	4
2 oz	soft margarine, melted	50 g
1 tsp	cajun seasoning	5 ml
2	medium onions, roughly chopped	2
2 tbsp	plain flour	30 ml
1 pt	skimmed milk	550 ml
1 tsp	dried mixed herbs	5 ml
8 oz	canned sweetcorn	225 g
1 oz	unsalted peanuts	25 g
	a pinch of cayenne pepper	

Brush the chicken portions with a little of the melted margarine and sprinkle with the cajun seasoning. Place on a baking tray and bake at 180°C (350°F) Gas Mark 4 for 1 hour, turning half way through cooking.

About 15 minutes before the end of cooking time, heat the remaining margarine in a saucepan. Add the onions and cook for 3-4 minutes. Stir in the flour and gradually blend in the milk. Bring to the boil, stirring constantly. Add the mixed herbs and stir in the sweetcorn. Transfer the chicken to a heat proof serving dish, pour the sauce over and sprinkle with the peanuts and cayenne pepper. Serve hot with brown rice and freshly cooked broccoli. Serves 4.

PER SERVING	
calories	371
g fat	17
g protein	30
g carbohydrate	26

A dish called Marengo is cooked in a sauce of mushrooms, tomatoes and garlic. It is said to have come from a dish that was cooked for Napoleon immediately after the battle of Marengo, 14th June 1800, from the only ingredients that were available.

Chicken Marengo

Use a large casserole dish to enable the chicken pieces to be browned more easily. As little oil is used to brown the chicken you may need to stir or turn the meat more frequently to prevent it sticking.

1 tbsp	plain flour	15 ml
4	medium boneless chicken breasts, skins removed	4
2 tbsp	olive or sunflower oil	30 ml
1	large onion, sliced	1
2	cloves garlic, crushed	2
4 oz	button mushrooms, wiped	100 g
2	cans (14 oz/400 g) chopped tomatoes	2
1/4 pt	chicken stock	150 ml
2 tbsp	brandy	30 ml
	salt and freshly ground black pepper	

Season the flour and use to coat the chicken breasts. Heat the oil in a large flameproof casserole dish and cook the chicken on both sides for 5-10 minutes until golden brown. Remove with a slotted spoon and reserve. Add the onion, garlic and mushrooms to the casserole and cook for 5 minutes until soft. Return the chicken to the casserole with the remaining ingredients. Season to taste. Bring to the boil, cover and simmer gently for 1 hour or until the chicken is cooked.

Transfer the chicken pieces to a warmed serving dish. If the sauce is too thin, boil briskly to reduce slightly and thicken. Spoon the sauce over the chicken and serve hot with freshly cooked brown rice or pasta. Serves 4.

PER SERVING	
calories	253
g fat	11
g protein	25
g carbohydrate	14

Fresh Mussels
When using fresh mussels, make sure that you discard any that are open or gaping before they are cooked and any that are not open after they are cooked.

Chicken, Spicy Sausage and Seafood Paella

There are many different versions of this popular Spanish dish. If you dislike mussels or find them difficult to prepare, use the same weight of firm white fish instead. Traditionally, saffron is used to colour and flavour this dish. Turmeric is very much cheaper but does not taste the same. Saffron is usually available in the spice section of the supermarket and you need only add a pinch in place of the turmeric for the authentic flavour.

2 tbsp	olive or corn oil	30 ml
1	large onion, finely chopped	1
2	cloves garlic, crushed	2
1	red pepper, deseeded and sliced	1
1	green pepper, deseeded and sliced	1
1 lb	boneless chicken breasts, skin removed and cut into 1-inch (2.5-cm) pieces	450 g
3 oz	chorizo sausage, sliced	75 g
1	can (8 oz/225 g) chopped tomatoes	1
8 oz	rice	225 g
2 tsp	turmeric	10 ml
1 pt	boiling chicken stock	550 ml
6 oz	fresh peeled prawns or thawed if frozen	175 g
6 oz	fresh mussels in shells, scrubbed	175 g
2 tbsp	chopped fresh parsley	30 ml

Heat the oil in a large wok or paella pan. Add the onion, garlic, peppers and chicken and cook for 5 minutes until soft. Add the sausage, tomatoes, rice, turmeric and stock. Stir well, bring to the boil, cover and simmer for 15 minutes. Stir the paella and cook uncovered for a further 15 minutes.

Add the prawns, mussels and parsley, bring back to the boil, and simmer uncovered for a further 5-10 minutes or until the mussels are cooked, the stock is absorbed and the rice is tender. The mussel shells should have opened. Discard any mussels that are not open. Serve immediately with crusty bread and a crisp green salad. Serves 4.

PER SERVING	
calories	618
g fat	23
g protein	51
g carbohydrate	54

Sauté of Lambs' Liver with Apple

This versatile dish can be served with potatoes and freshly cooked vegetables or with rice or pasta.

1 tbsp	plain flour	15 ml
	salt and freshly ground black pepper	
1 lb	sliced lambs' liver	450 g
2 tbsp	olive or sunflower oil	30 ml
1	medium onion, sliced	1
2	medium eating apples, cored and sliced	2
1 tsp	dry mustard	5 ml
1/4 pt	vegetable stock	150 ml
3 fl oz	unsweetened apple juice	75 ml

Season the flour and toss the liver in it to coat. Heat the oil in a large non-stick frying pan and cook the liver and onion for 4-5 minutes until the liver changes colour, stirring occasionally.

Add the apples to the pan and cook for 2-3 minutes, stirring. Stir in the remaining ingredients, bring to the boil and simmer for a further 5-10 minutes. Season to taste and serve with potatoes and freshly cooked vegetables. Serves 4.

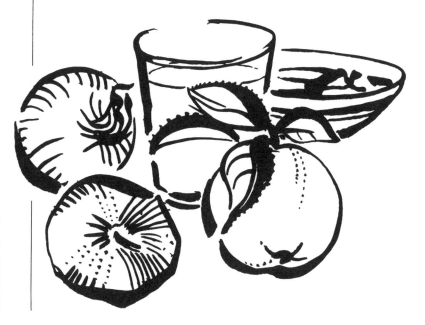

PER SERVING	
calories	325
g fat	20
g protein	24
g carbohydrate	15

A good curry should not have a watery sauce so cook uncovered for the last 15 minutes of cooking time until the sauce is well reduced and coating all the ingredients.

Indian Meal for 4
Cheese and Spinach Filo Triangles (page 35)
Lamb Rhogan (page 105)
served with rice
Pears with Ginger Sauce (page 169)

Lamb Rhogan

Use less curry powder if you prefer a milder taste as this provides a rather hot curry.

1 tbsp	olive or sunflower oil	15 ml
1¼ lb	lean lamb fillet, fat removed and cubed	550 g
1	large onion, sliced	1
2	cloves garlic, crushed	2
1 tbsp	hot curry powder	15 ml
1 tsp	turmeric	5 ml
½ pt	hot lamb stock	275 ml
1	can (14 oz/400 g) chopped tomatoes	1
4 oz	potato, peeled and diced	100 g
8 oz	carrots, diced	225 g
1 oz	sultanas	25 g

Heat the oil in a large saucepan, add the lamb, onion and garlic and cook for 5 minutes until browned. Stir in the curry powder and turmeric and cook for 1 minute, stirring continuously. Stir in the stock and tomatoes, cover and simmer for 40 minutes, or until the lamb is tender. Stir in the potato, carrot and sultanas. Cover and simmer for 15 minutes. Cook, uncovered for a further 15 minutes. Serve with freshly cooked brown rice. Serves 4.

PER SERVING	
calories	350
g fat	16
g protein	31
g carbohydrate	20

Wood pigeon are meaty little birds with a rich gamey flavour so one per person is ample. If you are buying them fresh from a game butcher or have been given them freshly shot look for feet that are supple and not scaly. This will indicate a tender young bird. They are, however, readily available oven ready in the chilled and frozen cabinets of most supermarkets.

Wood Pigeon with Walnuts

As wood pigeon are small birds, each person should have a whole one each.

1 tbsp	olive or sunflower oil	15 ml
4	wood pigeon	4
2	shallots, peeled and chopped	2
1 tbsp	cornflour	15 ml
2 tbsp	cold water	30 ml
1 pt	chicken stock	550 ml
1/4 pt	dry white wine	150 ml
3 oz	walnut halves, toasted	75 g
	salt and freshly ground black pepper	
2 tbsp	chopped fresh parsley	30 ml

Heat the oil in a flameproof casserole dish and brown the pigeon and shallots, stirring constantly. Mix the cornflour with the water and stir into the casserole with the stock and wine. Stir in the walnuts and season to taste. Bring to the boil, cover and transfer to a preheated oven at 160°C (325°F) Gas Mark 3 for 1 1/2 hours or until the pigeons are tender. Stir in parsley and adjust seasoning if necessary. Serve with wild rice and freshly cooked vegetables. Serves 4.

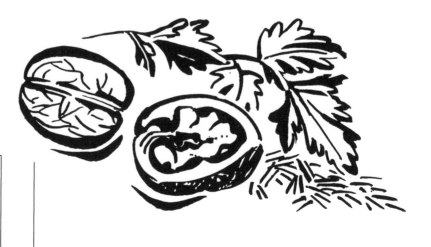

PER SERVING	
calories	474
g fat	32
g protein	34
g carbohydrate	9

Spanish Menu
*Chilled Summer Gazpacho
(page 27) served with fresh
crusty bread
Catalonian Chicken (page 107)
served with boiled rice
Spiced Apple Pie in Filo Pastry
(page 169)*

Catalonian Chicken

Chorizo sausages are usually located in the cold counter in
major supermarkets, alongside the cooked meats. If you prefer,
chicken breasts could be used instead of chicken quarters.

1 tbsp	plain flour	15 ml
	salt and freshly ground black pepper	
4	chicken quarters, skin removed	4
2 tbsp	olive or sunflower oil	30 ml
9 oz	shallots, skinned	250 g
2	cloves garlic, crushed	2
3/4 pt	hot chicken stock	425 ml
2 tbsp	dry white wine (optional)	30 ml
2 tbsp	tomato purée	30 ml
8 oz	button mushrooms, wiped	225 g
6 oz	cooked chorizo sausage, sliced	175 g

Season the flour and use to coat the chicken pieces. Heat the
oil in a large flameproof casserole dish and cook the chicken
until browned all over. Remove from the dish with a slotted
spoon and reserve.

Add the shallots and garlic to the casserole dish and cook for
5 minutes, until soft. Gradually stir in the stock, wine if using,
and tomato purée. Season to taste.

Cover and cook in a preheated oven at 180°C (350°F) Gas
Mark 4 for 1 hour. Add the mushrooms and chorizo sausage
and cook for a further 15 minutes, or until the chicken is tender.
Serves 4.

PER SERVING	
calories	421
g fat	32
g protein	28
g carbohydrate	7

Spicy Hungarian Goulash

I use my wok to cook this dish as even my largest saucepan isn't big enough. Goulash is traditionally a spicy dish, but you can vary the amount of paprika according to your taste. My husband and I both like spicy food so I used two tablespoons of hot paprika.

1 tbsp	olive or sunflower oil	15 ml
2 lb	lean braising steak, fat removed, cubed	900 g
2	onions, finely sliced	2
1-2 tbsp	paprika	15-30 ml
1 tbsp	plain flour	15 ml
1 tbsp	chopped fresh marjoram	15 ml
1 pt	hot beef stock	550 ml
	salt and freshly ground black pepper	
3 tbsp	sour cream	45 ml

Heat the oil in a large heavy-based saucepan. Add the meat and onions and cook for 4-5 minutes until brown. Stir in the paprika, flour and marjoram and cook for a further 2 minutes. Gradually stir in the stock and seasoning. Bring to the boil, reduce the heat, cover and simmer for $1\frac{1}{2}$ hours or until the meat is tender.

Spoon into warmed serving bowls and top with the soured cream. Sprinkle with a little paprika and serve with fresh crusty bread. Serves 4.

PER SERVING	
calories	450
g fat	18
g protein	65
g carbohydrate	7

Suitable for freezing.
Freeze after adding the cheese
sauce and before baking.
Defrost thoroughly and then
bake as in the recipe. Serve
with salads and crusty bread.

Make-Ahead Lasagne

When our daughter Jade was a baby, I found Lasagne was the
easiest dish to make for lunch when we had friends to stay.
I could prepare it well before they arrived so that I had more
time with our guests and Jade.

2	medium onions, finely chopped	2
1	clove garlic (optional)	1
1½ lb	lean mince	675 g
8 oz	mushrooms, sliced	225 g
1 tsp	dried oregano	5 ml
1 tsp	dried basil	5 ml
2 tbsp	tomato purée	30 ml
2	cans (14 oz/400 g) chopped tomatoes	2
¼ pt	boiling beef stock	150 ml
	salt and freshly ground black pepper	
1 oz	soft margarine	25 g
1 oz	plain flour	25 g
12 fl oz	skimmed milk	350 ml
4 oz	cheddar cheese, grated	100 g
8-9	sheets 'no-pre-cook' lasagne verdi	8-9

Place the onions, garlic (if using) mince and mushrooms in
a large non-stick pan and cook over a moderate heat for
5 minutes, until the meat is browned, stirring occasionally.
Drain off any excess fat. Add the herbs, tomato purée, tomatoes,
stock and season to taste. Stir well, bring to the boil, half cover
and simmer for 30 minutes, stirring occasionally until the sauce
is thickened and well reduced. Season to taste.

Meanwhile, make the cheese sauce. Place the margarine in a
saucepan with the flour and milk. Whisk continuously over a
moderate heat until thickened. Remove from the heat and stir in
1 oz (25 g) of the grated cheese. Season to taste.

Place half the meat sauce in the base of a large 4-pint (2-litre)
lasagne dish and cover with a layer of lasagne. Repeat with the
remaining meat sauce, finishing with a layer of lasagne. Pour
the cheese sauce over to cover the lasagne completely and
scatter the surface with the remaining cheese.

Cook in a preheated oven at 190°C (375°F) Gas Mark 5 for
40 minutes, or until golden brown and piping hot. Serve hot.
Serves 6.

PER SERVING	
calories	334
g fat	17
g protein	22
g carbohydrate	23

Chicory is a delicate vegetable that needs to be protected from the light to retain its white blanched colour. Most of the chicory now available is imported from Holland and Belgium and is packed in wooden crates and wrapped in dark blue tissue. Choose chicory that is crisp, firm and white with tightly packed leaves.

Chicory Gratin

This recipe comes from a French dish called 'Endives à l'ardennaise'. Chicory is known as endive in France.

8	chicory heads, cleaned and trimmed	8
1/4 pt	chicken stock	150 ml
4 tbsp	lemon juice	60 ml
3/4 pt	approx skimmed milk	425 ml
4	slices cooked lean ham, halved	4
1 oz	plain flour	25 g
1 oz	soft margarine	25 g
	salt and freshly ground black pepper	
3 oz	Gruyère cheese, grated	75 g

Cook the chicory in lightly salted boiling water for 5 minutes. Drain and place in a single layer in the base of a lightly greased ovenproof dish. Pour the chicken stock and lemon juice over, cover and bake in a preheated oven at 190°C (375°F) Gas Mark 5 for 1 hour.

Carefully remove the chicory from the dish and set aside. Pour the cooking juices into a measuring jug and add enough milk to make up to 1 pint (550 ml).

When the chicory is cool enough to handle, wrap a piece of ham around each and return to the ovenproof dish.

Make a white sauce by placing the stock and milk, flour and margarine in a saucepan. Season and whisk continuously over a moderate heat until thickened. Pour the sauce over the chicory. Sprinkle with the cheese and return to the oven for 15-20 minutes. Serve hot. Serves 4.

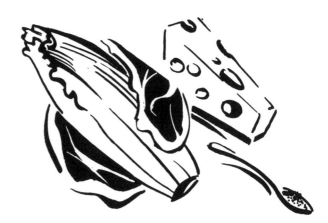

PER SERVING	
calories	243
g fat	15
g protein	15
g carbohydrate	12

Serve with boiled or mashed potatoes or Dry Roasted Potatoes (page 208) and freshly cooked green vegetables.

Casserole of Wood Pigeon

Wood pigeon are now commonly available ready prepared in main supermarkets in the game section of chilled cabinets.

2 tbsp	olive or sunflower oil	30 ml
4	oven-ready wood pigeons	4
2 oz	lean back bacon, rind removed and chopped	50 g
1	onion, chopped	1
1	clove garlic, crushed	1
2	large carrots, sliced	2
1 tbsp	plain flour	15 ml
1 tbsp	tomato purée	15 ml
3/4 pt	beef stock	425 ml
1 tsp	dried mixed herbs	5 ml
2	bay leaves	2
	salt and freshly ground black pepper	

Heat the oil in a large flameproof casserole dish and brown the pigeons on all sides. Remove with a slotted spoon and set aside. Add the bacon, onion, garlic and carrots to the casserole and cook for 5 minutes until the vegetables are soft. Stir in the flour and purée and cook for 1-2 minutes. Gradually stir in the stock. Add the mixed herbs and bay leaves. Season to taste. Return the pigeons to the casserole and bring the mixture to the boil. Cover and transfer to a preheated oven at 160°C (325°F) Gas Mark 3 for 1 1/2 hours. Serves 4.

PER SERVING	
calories	387
g fat	23
g protein	35
g carbohydrate	10

Tikka is a Hindi word that roughly translated means 'kebab'.

These skewered sticks of meat would also be ideal to cook on a barbecue.

Chicken Tikka

This comes from an authentic recipe from my brother's friend Mohammed. Serve with a side salad and freshly cooked boiled rice. If you are using wooden skewers, do soak them well in water before threading on the meat to prevent them burning during cooking.

1	carton (5 oz/150 g) low-fat natural yogurt	1
1 tbsp	ground ginger	15 ml
1 tbsp	chilli powder	15 ml
1 tbsp	ground coriander	15 ml
2 tsp	olive or sunflower oil	10 ml
2	cloves garlic, crushed	2
	a pinch of salt	
1 tsp	lemon juice	5 ml
4	medium boneless chicken breasts skin removed, cubed	4

Place the yogurt, spices, oil, garlic, salt and lemon juice in a bowl and mix well. Stir in the chicken and place in the refrigerator to marinate overnight.

Place the chicken cubes on to skewers and place under a preheated grill. Cook for 8-10 minutes, until cooked through, basting frequently with the marinade. Serve with boiled rice and a side salad. Serves 4.

PER SERVING	
calories	204
g fat	11
g protein	23
g carbohydrate	3

Pasta

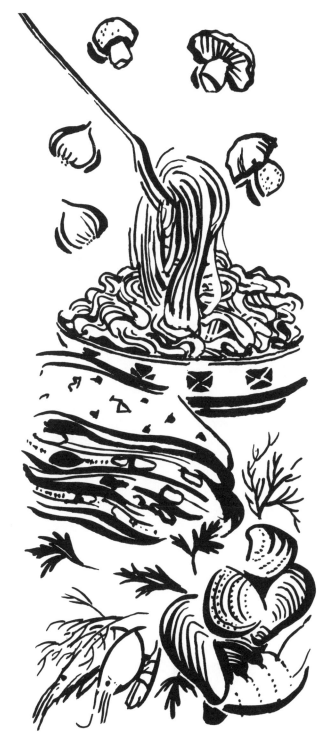

Pasta dishes are filling and economical as well as being a good source of starchy carbohydrate. Try experimenting with the different shapes and varieties. Some types are available in wholewheat which are higher in fibre, but any type of pasta is suitable for healthy eating, providing it is not smothered in high-fat sauces!

Serve with a crisp green salad and finish with fresh fruit for a delicious meal in minutes.

Spaghetti Tossed with Turkey and Walnuts

Turkey rashers are an alternative to bacon and are 98% fat free, with a saving of around 300 calories per 100 g! I've used 9 oz (250 g) of spaghetti which gives 40 g carbohydrate per serving. If you have a carbohydrate allowance per meal you can of course vary the amount of spaghetti/pasta to suit your needs – 2 oz (50 g) dry weight gives approximately 35 g carbohydrate.

9 oz	spaghetti	250 g
2 tsp	olive or sunflower oil	10 ml
2	5 oz (150 g) packets lean turkey rashers, chopped	2
1	clove of garlic, crushed	1
2 oz	walnuts, chopped	50 g
1	can (14 oz/400 g) chopped tomatoes	1
2 tbsp	freshly chopped parsley	30 ml
	freshly ground black pepper	

Cook the spaghetti in boiling salted water, according to the packet instructions until just tender.

Meanwhile, heat the oil in a medium-sized saucepan and sauté the turkey pieces, garlic and walnuts together until golden, stirring constantly. Stir in the tomatoes and parsley and heat, stirring continuously for 2-3 minutes until piping hot. Season with black pepper.

Drain the spaghetti and toss with the sauce. Serve immediately. Serves 4.

PER SERVING	
calories	395
g fat	13
g protein	22
g carbohydrate	50

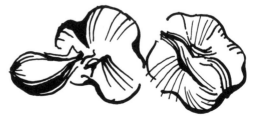

Serve with Tomato, Red Onion and Fresh Chive Salad (page 59).

Seafood Lasagne

Cod is naturally low in fat and makes a refreshing change to the more traditional meat lasagne.

12 oz	cod fillet	350 g
1¼ pt	skimmed milk	700 ml
2 oz	soft margarine	50 g
2 oz	plain flour	50 g
4 oz	peeled prawns	100 g
2 tbsp	chopped fresh parsley	30 ml
1	can (7 oz/200 g) sweetcorn, drained	1
2 tsp	lemon juice	10 ml
8	approx. sheets of no-pre-cook lasagne verdi	8
2 oz	cheddar, grated	50 g
	salt and freshly ground black pepper	

Place the fish and milk in a saucepan, cover and cook gently for 10-15 minutes. Reserving the cooking liquor, remove the fish and flake with a fork, removing any skin or bone. Place the margarine in a saucepan and melt over a low heat. Stir in the flour and cook for 1 minute. Gradually stir in the reserved milk and bring to the boil, stirring constantly until the sauce thickens. Remove from the heat and stir in the cod, prawns, parsley, sweetcorn and lemon juice. Season to taste.

Place half the lasagne over the base of a 9-inch (23-cm) square ovenproof dish. Cover with half the fish mixture. Repeat the layers once more, ending with a layer of sauce.

Sprinkle the grated cheese over the top and cook in a preheated oven at 180°C (350°F) Gas Mark 4 for 25-30 minutes or until golden brown. Serves 4-6.

PER SERVING	
calories	529
g fat	17
g protein	37
g carbohydrate	60

Chestnut Mushroom and Chicken Tagliatelle

Mushrooms are a very useful ingredient in a healthy diet. They add bulk to the dish allowing little or no meat to be used and they are delicious and 'meaty' in their own right. They are low in salt, have no cholesterol, carbohydrates or fat but are a good source of vegetable protein as well as important B-group vitamins and potassium.

12 oz	tagliatelle	350 g
1 tbsp	olive or corn oil	15 ml
1	small onion, finely chopped	1
1	clove garlic, crushed (optional)	1
8 oz	chestnut mushrooms, sliced	225 g
8 oz	cooked chicken, roughly chopped	225 g
2 tbsp	cornflour	30 ml
2 tbsp	cold water	30 ml
3/4 pt	boiling chicken stock	425 ml
1/4 pt	semi-skimmed milk	150 ml
	salt and freshly ground black pepper	

Cook the tagliatelle in boiling water according to the packet instructions until al dente. Drain in a colander.

Meanwhile, heat the oil in a non-stick frying pan or wok. Add the onion, garlic if using, and mushrooms and cook for 3-4 minutes until softened. Stir in the cooked chicken and cook for 1-2 minutes until browned. Mix the cornflour with the water and add to the pan, stirring continuously. Gradually stir in the hot stock and finally stir in the milk. Season to taste and stir until thickened. Serve spooned over the tagliatelle. Serves 4.

PER SERVING	
calories	460
g fat	8
g protein	25
g carbohydrate	78

Suitable for freezing – freeze before baking in the oven. Defrost thoroughly and bake as in the recipe.

Leafy Green Macaroni Cheese

Pasta dishes such as this recipe for macaroni cheese can provide the 'ideal' ratio of fat, carbohydrate and protein for healthy eating. This recipe has around 55% of calories from carbohydrate, 20% from fat and 20% from protein.

10 oz	macaroni	275 g
1 oz	soft margarine	25 g
1 oz	plain flour	25 g
3/4 pt	skimmed milk	425 ml
4 oz	cheddar, grated	100 g
8 oz	frozen chopped spinach, thawed	225 g
	freshly ground black pepper	

Cook the macaroni in boiling water according to the packet instructions until al dente and drain well.

Meanwhile, place the margarine, flour and milk in a saucepan and whisk continuously over a moderate heat until the sauce thickens. Remove from the heat and season to taste. Stir in half the cheese and all of the cooked macaroni. Drain the spinach and cook in a small saucepan for 3 minutes. Drain well and stir into the macaroni cheese mixture. Turn into a large ovenproof dish and sprinkle with the remaining grated cheese.

Bake in a preheated oven at 180°C (350°F) Gas Mark 4 for 20 minutes until the cheese topping is bubbling and golden brown. Serves 4.

PER SERVING	
calories	455
g fat	15
g protein	20
g carbohydrate	63

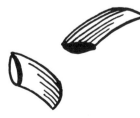

Suitable for freezing.
After adding the cheese sauce, cool quickly and freeze. Defrost thoroughly and then bake as in the recipe.

Oven-Baked Courgette, Red Pepper and Tuna Pasta

This recipe uses a fat-free white sauce which can also be used in other recipes which require a sauce.

8 oz	pasta	225 g
1 tbsp	olive or sunflower oil	15 ml
1	large onion, finely chopped	1
2	medium courgettes, sliced	2
1	large red pepper, deseeded and finely diced	1
1 tsp	dried mixed herbs	5 ml
1	can (7 oz/200 g) tuna in water or brine, drained	1

For the cheese sauce

2 tbsp	cornflour	30 ml
3/4 pt	skimmed milk	425 ml
3 oz	cheddar, grated	75 g
	salt and freshly ground black pepper	
	freshly chopped parsley to garnish	

Boil the pasta according to the packet instruction until tender, drain and set to one side.

Meanwhile, heat the oil in a non-stick frying pan and sauté the onion, courgette and pepper with the lid on for 4-5 minutes until soft. Stir in the mixed herbs, drained tuna and pasta and mix thoroughly. Turn into a large ovenproof dish.

Mix the cornflour with a little of the milk to form a smooth paste. Heat the remaining milk in a saucepan, then pour on to the cornflour mixture, stirring thoroughly.

Return the cornflour mixture to the saucepan, and stir continuously over a low heat for 1-2 minutes until thickened. Stir in the cheese and season to taste. Pour the cheese sauce over the pasta and bake at 200°C (400°F) Gas Mark 6 for 25 minutes until golden brown. Serve sprinkled with chopped fresh parsley. Serves 4-6.

PER SERVING	
calories	457
g fat	12
g protein	28
g carbohydrate	62

This could also be served as a tasty filling for a baked potato but if you have a carbohydrate allowance for each meal you will need to add the carbohydrate values for the potato or pasta that you serve with this sauce.

2 oz (50 g) dry weight of pasta gives approximately 35 g of carbohydrate or a 7 oz (200 g) jacket potato will give approximately 40 g of carbohydrate.

Gammon and Tomato Pasta Sauce

For a variation, thin strips of cooked pork or chicken could be used in place of the gammon.

2 tsp	olive or sunflower oil	10 ml
1	onion, finely chopped	1
1	clove garlic, crushed	1
1	can (14 oz/400 g) chopped tomatoes	1
1 tbsp	tomato purée	15 ml
3 tbsp	chopped fresh parsley	45 ml
2	thin cut gammon steaks, rind removed	2

Heat the oil in a saucepan, add the onion and garlic and cook for 5 minutes until soft, stirring occasionally. Stir in the tomatoes, purée and chopped parsley. Cover and simmer for 5 minutes until the sauce has thickened.

Meanwhile, cook the gammon steaks under a preheated grill for 15 minutes, turning occasionally, until cooked. Cut into cubes. Add the gammon to the tomato sauce and simmer for a further 5 minutes. Serve spooned over freshly cooked wholemeal pasta. Serves 2.

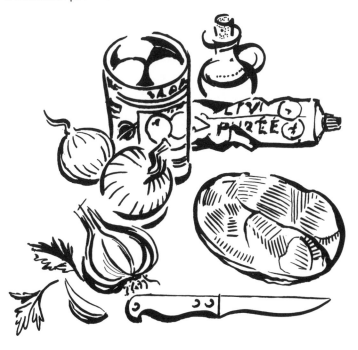

PER SERVING	
calories	260
g fat	10
g protein	34
g carbohydrate	8

Stir-Fried Shredded Pork and Pasta

Add some vegetables to the stir-fry if desired, such as green or red peppers, or baby sweetcorn. Serve with a crisp green salad. I've used 8 oz (225 g) of pasta which gives 35 g carbohydrate per serving. You can of course vary the amount of pasta to suit your needs and appetite – 2 oz (50 g) dry weight gives approximately 35 g carbohydrate.

1 lb	lean pork, diced and trimmed of fat	450 g
4 tbsp	white wine vinegar	60 ml
2 tbsp	soy sauce	30 ml
2 tbsp	tomato purée	30 ml
8 oz	pasta	225 g
1 tbsp	olive or corn oil	15 ml
2 tsp	cornflour	10 ml
2 tbsp	water	30 ml
8 oz	canned pineapple pieces in natural juice	225 g

Place the pork in a bowl and mix with the vinegar, soy sauce and tomato purée. Cover and marinate in the refrigerator for two hours. Cook the pasta in lightly salted boiling water for 8-10 minutes or according to the packet instructions. Meanwhile, drain the marinade mixture and reserve. Heat the oil in a non-stick frying pan or wok and stir-fry the pork for 4-5 minutes. Add the reserved marinade. Mix the cornflour with the water and add to the pan with the pineapple pieces and juice. Bring to the boil, stirring constantly, until the sauce thickens.

Drain the pasta and return to the hot pan. Stir in the pork and sauce. Toss together and serve immediately. Serves 4.

PER SERVING	
calories	439
g fat	13
g protein	32
g carbohydrate	54

Passata is sieved plum tomatoes and can be purchased from larger supermarkets. It makes an ideal base for a pasta sauce.

Chicken-Liver Pasta Sauce

Chicken livers are an excellent source of vitamin A needed for healthy skin and are also rich in iron and vitamin B12 needed for healthy blood. Spicy pork sausages or 'chorizo' can be found in delicatessen shops or in larger supermarkets.

2 tbsp	olive oil	30 ml
1 lb	chicken livers, chopped	450 g
1	large onion, finely chopped	1
4 oz	spicy pork sausages, chopped	100 g
1/2 pt	Passata	275 ml
1/4 pt	chicken stock	150 ml
	salt and freshly ground black pepper	
3 tbsp	freshly chopped parsley	45 ml

Heat the oil in a non-stick frying pan with lid, and cook the chicken livers and onion for 3-4 minutes over a moderate heat, stirring frequently. Add the sausages and cook for 1-2 minutes, stirring occasionally.

Stir in the passata and stock and bring to the boil. Cover and simmer for 10-15 minutes. Season and stir in the chopped parsley. Serve with freshly cooked pasta. Serves 4.

PER SERVING	
calories	272
g fat	17
g protein	25
g carbohydrate	5

Ten-Minute Carbonara

Friends often say they would like some recipes which can be quickly prepared when they get home from work. Well this is ideal as it takes very little preparation. Serve with a crisp salad, and fresh crusty bread if desired.

10 oz	spaghetti	275 g
6 oz	lean back bacon, derinded	175 g
4 oz	mushrooms, sliced	100 g
5 fl oz	half-fat single cream	150 ml
1	egg, beaten	1
1 oz	cheddar, grated	25 g
2 tbsp	chopped fresh parsley	30 ml
8 oz	cooked lean chicken, cut into strips	225 g
	salt and freshly ground black pepper	

Cook the spaghetti in a large pan in lightly salted boiling water for 8-10 minutes or until al dente. Meanwhile, grill the bacon until crisp. Snip into pieces. Add the mushrooms to the spaghetti 2 minutes before the end of cooking time. Beat the cream, egg, cheese and parsley together. Drain the spaghetti and return to the hot pan. Stir in the bacon, chicken, cream mixture and seasoning. Toss together over a medium heat until hot and the sauce thickens. Serve immediately. Serves 4.

PER SERVING	
calories	452
g fat	14
g protein	34
g carbohydrate	52

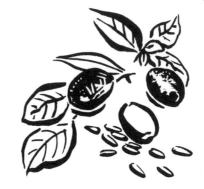

Red Pesto Pasta

Pesto sauce can be brought ready made in jars, but it is easy to make at home and you benefit from the delicious aroma and taste of fresh basil.

1	packet (¹/₂ oz/15 g) fresh basil leaves, chopped	1
1	clove garlic, crushed	1
1 oz	pine nuts	25 g
2 oz	fresh Parmesan, grated	50 g
1	jar (11 oz/300 g) sun-dried tomatoes, in olive oil	1
14 oz	pasta	400 g
4 oz	black olives, pitted	100 g

If you cannot get fresh basil leaves, look for jars of freshly chopped basil in the spice section of the supermarket.

Place the basil, garlic, and pine nuts in a food processor or liquidiser. Process for a few seconds. Add the parmesan and process for a few more seconds. Add half the tomatoes, with all of the olive oil and blend for a few seconds more, to form a smooth paste.

Cook the pasta in boiling water according to the packet instructions until al dente. Drain and toss together with the pesto sauce, olives and remaining tomatoes. Serve immediately with a freshly made salad. Serves 6.

PER SERVING	
calories	470
g fat	25
g protein	24
g carbohydrate	51

Right:
Quick Grilled Salmon with Garlic and Peppercorns
(page 50)

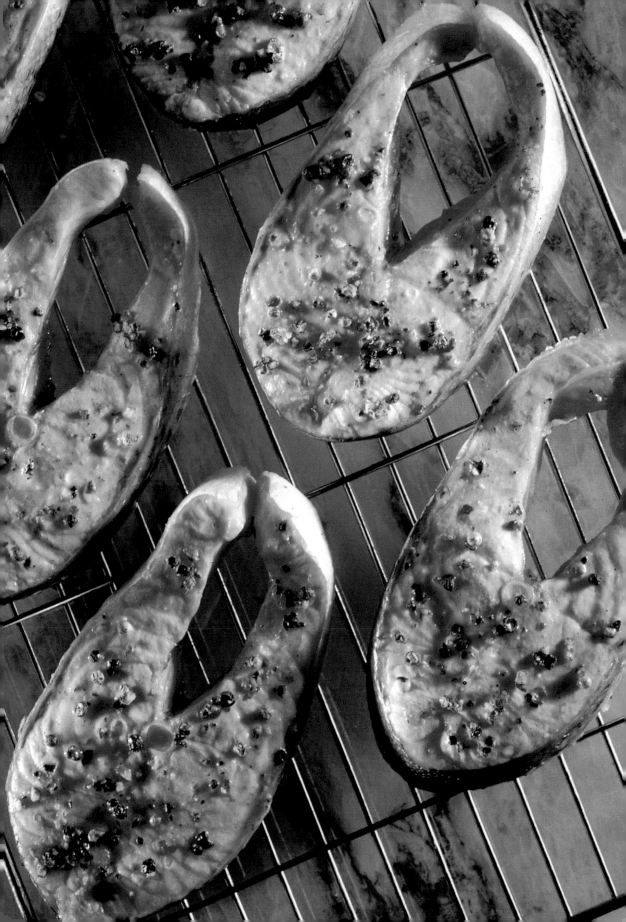

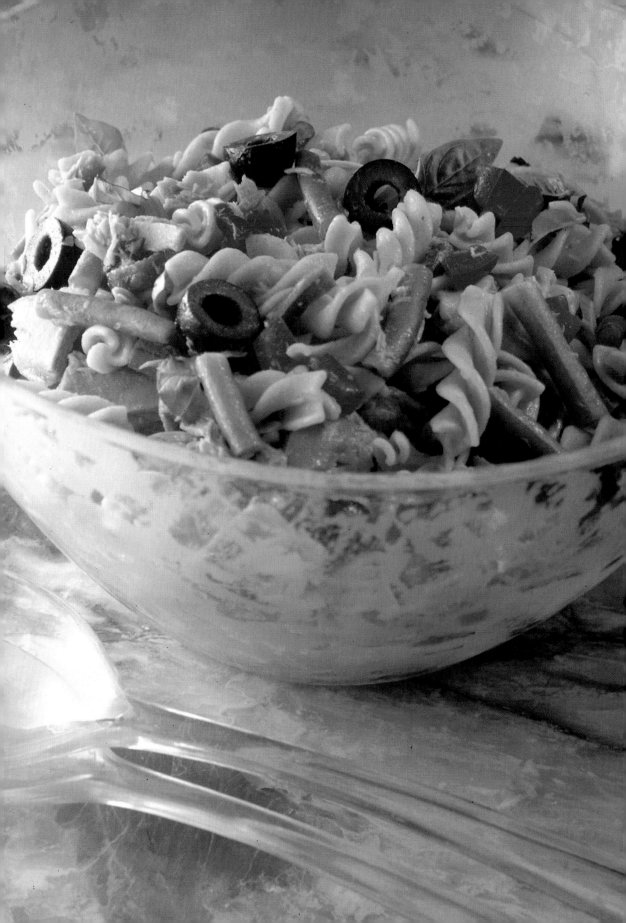

Yellow Split Pea and Turkey Pasta Sauce

Using split peas means that less meat is needed for this dish as they are both filling and a valuable source of soluble fibre. Remember to soak the split peas overnight before cooking. Minced turkey is available fresh or frozen. Be sure to defrost frozen mince thoroughly before use.

4 oz	split yellow peas	100 g
8 oz	lean minced turkey	225 g
1	large onion, finely chopped	1
1	clove garlic, crushed	1
3/4 pt	chicken or vegetable stock	425 ml
1	can (14 oz/400 g) chopped tomatoes	1
2 tbsp	tomato purée	30 ml
	salt and freshly ground black pepper	

Soak the split peas overnight in plenty of cold water. Rinse thoroughly and place in a saucepan with fresh water. Bring to the boil and boil rapidly for 10 minutes. Rinse and drain. Place the turkey, onion and garlic in a non-stick pan and cook over a moderate heat for 3-4 minutes, stirring. Add the drained split peas and cook for 1-2 minutes, stirring occasionally. Add the remaining ingredients and mix well. Season to taste. Bring to the boil, cover and simmer for 30-40 minutes. Serve with freshly cooked pasta and a crisp salad. Serves 4.

PER SERVING	
calories	161
g fat	2
g protein	20
g carbohydrate	19

Left
Red Pepper, Basil and Tuna
Pasta Salad (page 40)

You can substitute a raw cured ham such as Prosciutto or Parma ham in this recipe for an even speedier result.

Classic Carbonara

A classic pasta dish which is quick to prepare for supper or lunch.

6 oz	spaghetti	175 g
6	rashers lean back bacon, fat removed and cut into thin strips	6
2	size 3 eggs	2
1 tbsp	chopped fresh parsley	15 ml
	salt and freshly ground black pepper	
1 oz	freshly grated Parmesan cheese	25 g

Cook the spaghetti in boiling water according to the packet instructions, until al dente. Dry fry the bacon in a non-stick frying pan until crisp and brown, stirring frequently. Drain on kitchen paper.

Beat the eggs, stir in the parsley and season to taste. Drain the spaghetti, return to the hot pan, but remove from the heat. Add the egg mixture and stir well until the eggs set slightly. Sprinkle the bacon and cheese on top and toss well. Spoon into warm serving bowls and serve at once with a crisp green salad. Serves 2.

PER SERVING	
calories	536
g fat	17
g protein	36
g carbohydrate	65

Baking

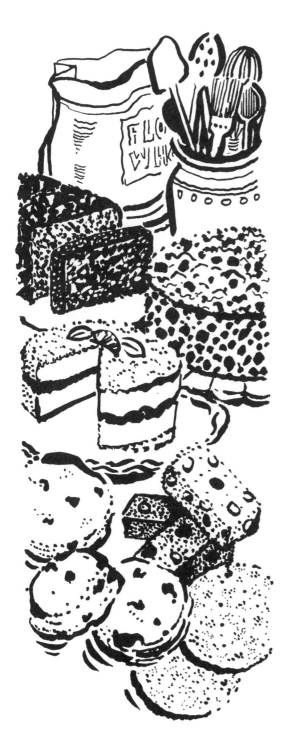

Many people are concerned that they will be unable to eat cakes and biscuits once they have been diagnosed with diabetes. However, it is still possible to have these occasionally as part of an overall healthy diet. The recipes in this section have been developed using less fat and sugar where possible. Some recipes have no added sugar but rely upon the natural sweetness of dried fruit. Because of the reduced sugar and fat content, the cakes and biscuits are best eaten within a few days or alternatively they may be frozen in convenient portions and used as required. This will ensure that they are eaten at their best.

Best eaten within 2 days.
Suitable for freezing.

An excellent way to use up
bananas when they have started
to get too soft to enjoy raw.

Banana Loaf

The dates add bulk to the mixture and replace the sugar and fat
usually required in a cake recipe. Why not try replacing the
sugar in some of your own recipes with a date purée? Dates
contain around half the carbohydrate and calories as the same
weight of sugar. (See page 139.)

6 oz	stoned dried dates	175 g
4 fl oz	water	100 ml
1	egg	1
8 oz	self-raising wholemeal flour	225 g
1 tsp	ground mixed spice	5 ml
1 lb	ripe bananas, peeled	450 g
4 oz	chopped walnuts	100 g

Grease and base-line a 2 lb (900 g) loaf tin. Place the dates
and water in a saucepan and simmer gently until the dates are
soft. Mash with a fork until the dates are puréed. Allow to cool
slightly. Beat in the egg. Mix together the flour and spice.
Mash the bananas until smooth, then stir into the date mixture
with the flour and spice. Stir in the walnuts.

Spoon the mixture into the prepared tin and level the surface.
Bake in a preheated oven at 180°C (350°F) Gas Mark 4 for
1 hour or until a skewer when inserted in the centre comes out
clean. Cover with foil if becoming too brown.

Allow to cool in the tin for 15 minutes before turning out on
a wire rack to cool completely. Serve sliced. Makes 14 slices.

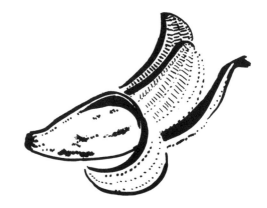

PER SLICE	
calories	164
g fat	6
g protein	4
g carbohydrate	25

Best eaten within 2 days.
Suitable for freezing.

Carrot and Banana Squares

This recipe is quick to make and would be useful in packed lunch boxes or as a snack.

10 oz	self-raising wholemeal flour	275 g
1½ tsp	baking powder	7.5 ml
1 tsp	mixed spice	5 ml
2 oz	porridge oats	50 g
2 oz	light soft brown sugar	50 g
2	small bananas, peeled and mashed	2
8 oz	carrots, peeled and finely grated	225 g
4	eggs, beaten	4
3 fl oz	olive or sunflower oil	75 ml
	a few drops of vanilla essence	

Sift the flour, baking powder and spice into a bowl, tipping any bran remaining in the sieve back into the bowl. Stir in the oats and sugar. Add the remaining ingredients and beat well with a wooden spoon. Pour into a lightly greased 11 x 9-inch (28 x 23-cm) tin. Bake in a preheated oven at 180°C (350°F) Gas Mark 4 for 40-50 minutes, or until a skewer inserted into the centre comes out clean. Leave to cool in the tin for a few minutes, then turn out on to a wire rack to cool completely. Cut into squares. Makes 24 squares.

PER SQUARE	
calories	131
g fat	5
g protein	4
g carbohydrate	18

Suitable for freezing.
I cut cakes into slices before freezing so that individual pieces may be taken out when required. These fingers are ideal to include in lunch boxes as a snack.

Coconut and Cherry Fingers

These fingers will keep for up to two days in an airtight tin or alternatively they may be frozen.

8 oz	plain flour	225 g
2 tsp	baking powder	10 ml
4 oz	soft margarine	100 g
1 oz	caster sugar	25 g
2 oz	desiccated coconut	50 g
4 oz	glacé cherries, washed, dried and chopped	100 g
1	egg, beaten	1
2 tbsp	lemon juice	30 ml
7 fl oz	skimmed milk	200 ml

Sift the flour and baking powder together in a large bowl. Rub in the margarine until the mixture resembles breadcrumbs. Stir in the sugar, coconut and cherries. Stir in the egg and lemon juice and enough milk to mix to a soft dropping consistency. Spoon into a lightly greased and base-lined 11 x 7-inch (28 x 18-cm) shallow tin. Bake in a preheated oven at 160°C (325°F) Gas Mark 3 for 40-45 minutes or until golden brown and firm. Turn out on to a wire rack. Cut into fingers when cold. Makes 16.

PER FINGER	
calories	146
g fat	7
g protein	3
g carbohydrate	18

Quick Chocolate Squares

These squares could be decorated with a little icing (see page 152) for a children's party.

1 tbsp	cocoa powder, sifted	15 ml
2 tbsp	boiling water	30 ml
8 oz	plain flour	225 g
2 tsp	baking powder	10 ml
6 oz	soft margarine	175 g
3 oz	caster sugar	75 g
3	eggs, beaten	3
3 tbsp	skimmed or semi-skimmed milk	45 ml

Stir the cocoa powder and the boiling water together until smooth. Sift the flour and baking powder together and beat in the cocoa mixture with the margarine, sugar, eggs and milk. Beat until smooth. Spoon into a lightly greased and base-lined 11 x 9-inch (28 x 23-cm) tin. Bake in a preheated oven at 180°C (350°F) Gas Mark 4 for 25-30 minutes. Cool in the tin, before turning out on to a wire rack to cool completely. Cut into 20 squares.

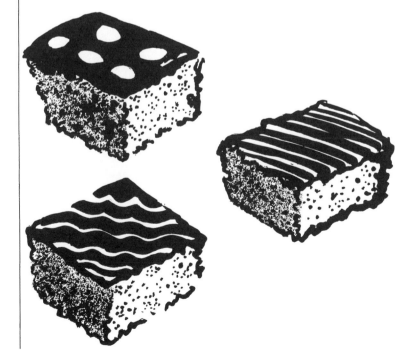

PER SQUARE	
calories	131
g fat	8
g protein	3
g carbohydrate	11

Muffins can make a delicious treat for a lazy weekend breakfast. Serve with fresh fruit for a substantial start to the day with tea or coffee and the newspapers.

Sultana Nut Muffins

Muffins are usually very high in calories. However, by cutting down on the fat and sugar content and increasing the fibre by using wholemeal flour, these muffins are both nutritious and tasty to eat.

6 oz	plain wholemeal flour	175 g
4 oz	plain flour	100 g
1/2 tsp	salt	2.5 ml
2 tbsp	baking powder	30 ml
1 oz	caster sugar	25 g
4 oz	soft margarine, melted	100 g
2	eggs	2
9 fl oz	skimmed milk	250 ml
2 tsp	vanilla essence	10 ml
3 oz	sultanas	75 g
2 oz	flaked almonds	50 g

Sift the flours, salt and baking powder into a large bowl, tip any bran remaining in the sieve back into the bowl.

In another bowl, mix together the sugar, melted margarine, eggs, milk and vanilla essence. Spoon in the flour mixture and add the sultanas and half the almonds. Using a large metal spoon, stir to bring the mixture together quickly. Don't over-beat or the muffins will be heavy.

Line a muffin tin with 12 muffin cases. Spoon the mixture evenly into the paper cases. Sprinkle the remaining almonds over the tops. Bake in a preheated oven at 200°C (400°F) Gas Mark 6 for 25 minutes, or until well risen and golden. Serve warm, or cool slightly and dust with a little granulated artificial sweetener if desired before serving. Makes 12.

PER SERVING	
calories	208
g fat	11
g protein	6
g carbohydrate	24

Spiced Apple and Almond Cake

This cake will keep for up to 3 days but it is suitable for freezing. Cut into slices when freezing if you want to be able to take out individual slices when required.

1¼ lb	eating apples, peeled, cored and roughly chopped	550 g
1 tbsp	lemon juice	15 ml
3 tbsp	water	45 ml
4 oz	self-raising flour	100 g
2 tsp	baking powder	10 ml
8 oz	soft margarine	225 g
3 oz	soft light brown sugar	75 g
4	eggs, size 2, beaten	4
½ tsp	almond essence	2.5 ml
1 oz	ground almonds	25 g
1½ tsp	ground cinnamon	7.5 ml

Place the apples in a saucepan with the lemon juice and water. Cook over a gentle heat until just beginning to soften – there shouldn't be any liquid left. Leave to cool. Place the remaining ingredients in a food processor with half the apple mixture. Blend for a few seconds until smooth. Pour half the cake mixture into a greased and base-lined 8-inch (20-cm) round tin. Spoon the remaining apples over and carefully top with the remaining cake mixture to cover the apple completely. Bake in a preheated oven at 180°C (350°F) Gas Mark 4 for 50-60 minutes or until a skewer when inserted in the centre comes out clean. Cool in the tin for 5 minutes before turning out on to a wire rack to cool completely. Cut into slices. Makes 16 slices.

PER SLICE	
calories	214
g fat	14
g protein	4
g carbohydrate	18

Best eaten within 1-2 days.
Suitable for freezing.

Apricot Pecan Slice

This could also be served as a dessert, with a little half-fat cream or custard.

6 oz	plain wholemeal flour	175 g
6 oz	plain flour	175 g
1 tbsp	baking powder	15 ml
2 tsp	cinnamon	10 ml
3 oz	caster sugar	75 g
2 oz	soft margarine	50 g
2	eggs, beaten	2
1/4 pt	skimmed milk	150 ml
1	can (14 oz/400 g) apricots in natural juice, drained and chopped	1
4 oz	pecan nuts, chopped	100 g
1	orange, grated rind	1

Sift together the flours, baking powder and cinnamon into a large bowl. Tip any bran remaining in the sieve back into the bowl. Stir in the sugar. Add the margarine, eggs and milk and stir gently until smooth. Do not beat. Fold in the chopped apricots, nuts and grated orange rind. Pour into a 11 x 7-inch (23 x 18-cm) lightly greased and base-lined tin. Bake in a preheated oven at 180°C (350°F) Gas Mark 4 for 40 minutes until golden, or when a skewer when inserted comes out clean. Cool in the tin and cut into 16 slices.
Makes 16 slices.

PER SLICE	
calories	177
g fat	8
g protein	5
g carbohydrate	22

This is a delicious way to use up bread that is no longer perfectly fresh!

Bread Pudding

7 oz	wholemeal breadcrumbs	200 g
1/4 pt	warm skimmed milk	150 ml
7 oz	mixed dried fruit such as sultanas, currants	200 g
2 tbsp	sugar	30 ml
1/2 oz	soft margarine	15 g
2 tsp	ground mixed spice	10 ml
1	small carrot, peeled and finely grated	1
1	egg, beaten	1

Place the bread in a bowl, cover with the warm milk and leave to soak for 30 minutes. Beat the bread until smooth, then stir in the dried fruit, sugar, margarine and spice. Stir in the carrot and egg and beat to give a soft consistency. Pour the mixture into a lightly greased shallow 2-pt (1-litre) ovenproof dish. Bake in a preheated oven at 180°C (350°F) Gas Mark 4 for 45 minutes, or until golden brown. Cool in the dish and cut into 12.

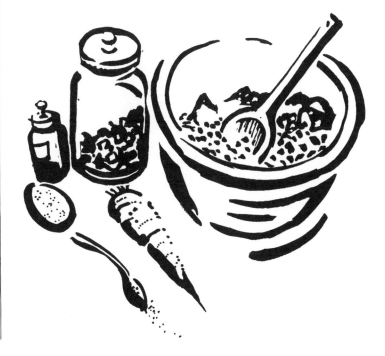

PER SLICE	
calories	105
g fat	2
g protein	3
g carbohydrate	20

Best eaten within 1-2 days.
Suitable for freezing.

Oat and Ginger Cookies

Sprinkle the cookies with a little granulated artificial sweetener when cooked if you prefer a sweeter taste.

5 oz	soft margarine	150 g
2 oz	caster sugar	50 g
1	egg, beaten	1
3 oz	rolled oats	75 g
5 oz	plain flour	150 g
1/2 tsp	baking powder	2.5 ml
1/2 tsp	salt	2.5 ml
1 1/2 tsp	ground ginger	7.5 ml
1 tsp	vanilla essence	5 ml

Beat together all the ingredients until combined. Place in spoonfuls, spaced apart on to lightly greased baking sheets. Flatten slightly with a fork. Bake in a preheated oven at 190°C (375°F) Gas Mark 5 for 10-15 minutes, or until golden and just firm to the touch. Cool on a wire rack. Makes approximately 26.

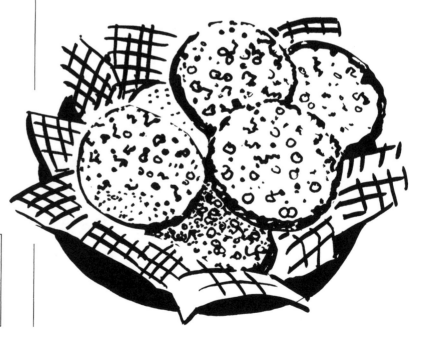

PER COOKIE	
calories	82
g fat	5
g protein	1
g carbohydrate	7

Date and Apricot Bars

When I asked my nieces to try these out for me, their comments were: Amy (age 7) 'Mmm-nice' and from Katie (age 9) 'Lovely, scrummy, yummy'. And mum said 'can I have the recipe please'! They would be useful to have before exercise.

6 oz	stoned dates, chopped	175 g
4 oz	ready-to-eat dried apricots, chopped	100 g
1/4 pt	water	150 ml
9 oz	soft margarine	250 g
1 oz	soft brown sugar	25 g
6 oz	plain wholemeal flour	175 g
1 tsp	baking powder	5 ml
7 oz	rolled oats	200 g

Place the dates and apricots in a saucepan with the water and simmer for 10 minutes until soft and the mixture forms a paste. Melt the margarine and sugar in a saucepan. Remove from the heat and stir in the flour, baking powder and oats. Press half the mixture into the base of a lightly greased 9 x 11-inch (23 x 28-cm) shallow tin. Spoon the date and apricot mixture over the top. Spoon the remaining oat mixture over to cover evenly and press down (I use my fingers). Bake in a preheated oven at 180°C (350°F) Gas Mark 4 for 30 minutes until evenly browned.

Allow to cool in the tin for 10 minutes. Mark into 16 bars and cool completely on a wire rack. Makes 16.

PER BAR	
calories	224
g fat	14
g protein	3
g carbohydrate	23

Store in an airtight tin. Suitable for freezing.

These days everyone should be trying to eat a low-fat, high-fibre diet so don't keep these recipes for yourself. If you need to contribute to a cake stall, label this cake as 'Healthy Eating' and watch it get snapped up.

Lemon Sesame Cake

This is ideal if you prefer a plainer type of cake. It is best eaten within 2-3 days.

4 oz	soft margarine	100 g
2 oz	caster sugar	50 g
2	size 2 eggs, beaten	2
8 oz	self-raising flour	225 g
1	carton (5 oz/150 g) low-fat natural yogurt	1
2 tbsp	sesame seeds	30 ml
1	large lemon, grated rind and juice	1

Cream the margarine and sugar together, then gradually beat in the eggs. Sift the flour. Fold in with the yogurt and mix well. Lastly, fold in the sesame seeds, grated lemon rind and juice. Place in a greased and base-lined 2 lb (900 g) loaf tin and level the surface.

Bake in a preheated oven at 160°C (325°F) Gas Mark 3 for approximately 1 hour until risen and firm to the touch. Cool on a wire rack. Decorate with lemon slices if desired. Cuts into 14 slices.

PER SLICE	
calories	148
g fat	9
g protein	4
g carbohydrate	15

Suitable for freezing.

Lemon and Almond Cake

The sliced lemons on top of the cake give an attractive finish.
I found the combination of lemons and almonds very refreshing
compared to traditional recipes of this type which tend to be
very sweet.

6 oz	soft margarine	175 g
3 oz	caster sugar	75 g
3	eggs, beaten	3
6 oz	self-raising flour	150 g
1/2 tsp	baking powder	2.5 ml
2 oz	ground almonds	50 g
1	large lemon, grated rind and juice	1
1/2 tsp	almond essence	2.5 ml
To finish		
2	lemons	2
1 tbsp	marmalade	15 ml
1 tbsp	water	15 ml

Place all the cake ingredients in a large bowl. Mix well and
beat with a wooden spoon or electric mixer for 2-3 minutes
until light and fluffy. Turn the mixture into a lightly greased and
base-lined 8-inch (20-cm) loose-bottomed, round cake tin.
Smooth the top.

Pare the rind and pith from the two lemons, then slice the
flesh into thin rounds. Arrange on top of the cake.

Bake in a preheated oven at 160°C (325°F) Gas Mark 3 for
50-60 minutes until golden and firm. Cool in the tin for 5
minutes, then release the sides and cool on a wire rack.

Warm the marmalade and water together. Sieve and brush
over the top of the cake whilst still warm. Cuts into 14 slices.

PER SLICE	
calories	190
g fat	14
g protein	4
g carbohydrate	14

They are best eaten the same day or may be frozen.

Farmhouse Fruit Scones

You may need to use all of the egg and milk if the mixture seems dry as this will vary with the flour used. Use a little extra milk for brushing the tops of the scones before baking.

8 oz	plain flour	225 g
2½ tsp	baking powder	12.5 ml
½ tsp	salt	2.5 ml
2 oz	soft margarine	50 g
1 oz	caster sugar	25 g
2 oz	sultanas	50 g
1	egg, beaten with sufficient skimmed milk to make ¼ pt (150 ml) liquid	1

Sift the flour, baking powder and salt together, tipping any bran remaining in the sieve back into the bowl. Rub in the margarine until the mixture resembles breadcrumbs. Stir in the sugar and sultanas. Gradually add enough of the egg and milk mixture to form a soft dough.

Knead the mixture on a lightly floured surface and roll out to approximately ½-inch (1-cm) thickness. Cut into 2-inch (5-cm) rounds, rerolling the trimmings. Place on a floured baking sheet and brush the tops with a little extra milk if required. Bake in a preheated oven at 220°C (425°F) Gas Mark 7 for 10-12 minutes. Cool on a wire rack. Makes approximately 14.

PER SCONE	
calories	99
g fat	4
g protein	3
g carbohydrate	15

Unfortunately, due to the reduced sugar and fat content this cake is best eaten within 1-2 days, or alternatively it may be frozen.

Ginger and Date Cake

Dried dates are naturally sweet and therefore no extra sugar is added to this cake. Puréed dates can be used to replace some or all of the sugar in some cakes.

4 fl oz	skimmed milk	100 ml
5 oz	dried stoned dates, roughly chopped	150 g
1 tsp	bicarbonate of soda	5 ml
8 oz	plain wholemeal flour	225 g
2 tsp	baking powder	10 ml
2 tsp	ground ginger	10 ml
1 tsp	ground cinnamon	5 ml
4 oz	soft margarine	100 g
1 oz	ground almonds	25 g
3	eggs, beaten	3
2 tbsp	water	30 ml

Place the milk and dates in a saucepan and heat gently for 5 minutes until the dates are soft. Stir in the bicarbonate of soda and set aside.

Sift together the flour, baking powder and spices, tipping any bran remaining in the sieve back into the bowl. Rub in the margarine until the mixture resembles fine breadcrumbs. Stir in the ground almonds. Gradually beat in the beaten eggs and finally stir in the water and date mixture. Beat well to combine. Place the mixture into a lightly greased and base-lined 2 lb (900 g) loaf tin and level the surface.

Bake in a preheated oven at 180°C (350°F) Gas Mark 4 for 35-40 minutes until the cake is risen and a skewer inserted into the centre comes out clean. Cool on a wire rack. Cuts into 14 slices.

PER SLICE	
calories	146
g fat	9
g protein	4
g carbohydrate	14

Wrap well and store in an airtight container. It will keep for 3-4 days or alternatively it can be frozen.

Apricot and Sultana Loaf

A moist fruit loaf which is high in fibre (3 g per slice) and low in fat.

4 oz	All-bran cereal	100 g
4 oz	dried ready-to-eat apricots, chopped	100 g
4 oz	sultanas	100 g
½ pt	strong hot tea	275 ml
3 oz	self-raising wholemeal flour	75 g
2	eggs, beaten	2

Place the All-bran, apricots, sultanas and tea in a bowl and mix well. Leave to stand for 15-20 minutes. Stir in the flour and eggs and mix well. Place in a lightly greased and base-lined 2 lb (900 g) loaf tin and level the surface.

Bake in a preheated oven at 180°C (350°F) Gas Mark 4 for approximately 45-50 minutes, or until a skewer inserted in the centre comes out clean. Allow to cool on a wire rack. Cuts into 14 slices.

PER SLICE	
calories	70
g fat	2
g protein	3
g carbohydrate	12

Brenda's Boiled Fruit Cake

This recipe was given to me by my mother and I have adapted it to make it more in line with healthy eating dietary guidelines.

9 fl oz	water	250 ml
1 oz	sugar	25 g
4 oz	soft margarine	100 g
1/2 tsp	mixed spice	2.5 ml
1/2 tsp	bicarbonate of soda	2.5 ml
1 lb	mixed dried fruit	450 g
2	size 2 eggs, beaten	2
8 oz	self-raising wholemeal flour	225 g

Place the water, sugar, margarine, mixed spice, bicarbonate of soda and dried fruit in a medium-sized saucepan. Boil together for 5 minutes, stirring occasionally, remove from the heat and set aside to cool.

When cooked, stir in the eggs and flour and beat well. Turn into a greased and base-lined 9-inch (23-cm) cake tin and level the surface. Bake in a preheated oven at 160°C (325°F) Gas Mark 3 for 1 hour, or until a skewer when inserted comes out clean. Cuts into 20 small slices.

PER SLICE	
calories	147
g fat	5
g protein	3
g carbohydrate	24

Best eaten within 1-2 days.
Suitable for freezing.
Store in an airtight container.

All-in-One Madeira Cake

6 oz	soft margarine	175 g
3 oz	caster sugar	75 g
3	eggs, beaten	3
7 oz	plain flour	200 g
1½ tsp	baking powder	7.5 ml
	finely grated rind of half a lemon	

Place all the ingredients in a bowl and beat with a wooden spoon until well mixed (approx 2-3 minutes). Place in a lightly greased and base-lined deep 7-inch (18-cm) cake tin and level the top. Bake in a preheated oven at 160°C (325°F) Gas Mark 3 for 1-1¼ hours, or until a skewer when inserted comes out clean. Allow to cool in the tin for a few minutes before turning out to cool on a wire rack. Cuts into 16 slices.

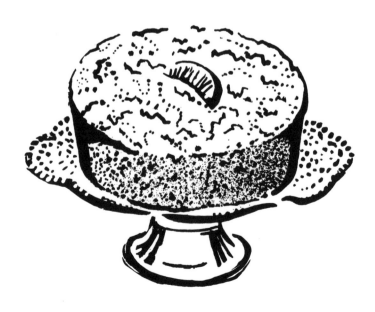

PER SLICE	
calories	158
g fat	10
g protein	3
g carbohydrate	15

Best eaten within 1-2 days.
Suitable for freezing.
Store in an airtight container.

Jiffy Jammy Roll

A Swiss roll is a low-fat cake that is quick to make and quick to bake. Working swiftly gives the best result too when you are rolling the cake. If it is allowed to cool, it cracks more easily so have everything ready to hand before you take it out of the oven.

3	eggs	3
3 oz	caster sugar	75 g
4 oz	plain flour	100 g
1 tbsp	warm water	15 ml
2 tsp	caster sugar for dredging	10 ml
4 tbsp	jam, warmed	60 ml

Place the eggs and sugar in a large mixing bowl. Place the bowl over a pan of gently simmering water and whisk until thick and creamy. (Alternatively, use an electric food mixer.) The whisk should leave a trail in the mixture when lifted. Remove from the heat. Sift the flour, then lightly sieve into the egg mixture. Fold in carefully with the water using a figure of eight movement. Pour the mixture into a lightly greased and lined 13 x 9-inch (32.5 x 23-cm) Swiss roll tin, tapping the mixture into the corners of the tin until it evenly covers the surface. Bake in a preheated oven at 220°C (425°F) Gas Mark 7 for 8-10 minutes or until well risen and the cake springs back when lightly touched with a finger tip.

Have ready a large sheet of greaseproof paper, sprinkled with caster sugar. Place the paper on a clean tea-towel, wrung out in hot water (this will make it easier to roll up). Turn the cooked sponge out on to the greaseproof paper and remove the lining paper. Trim off the crusty edges with a sharp knife. Make a crease in the short side of the sponge with the back of a knife and roll up the sponge and greaseproof paper firmly. Leave on a wire rack to cool. When cold, carefully unroll. Spread with the warmed jam and re-roll the sponge. Serve sliced. Cuts into 10.

PER SLICE	
calories	106
g fat	2
g protein	3
g carbohydrate	20

Best eaten within 2 days.
Suitable for freezing.
Wrap well in foil and store in an airtight tin or container.

Old Fashioned Gingerbread

As the sugar has been greatly reduced in this recipe, it will not taste as sweet as traditional sticky gingerbread but I think I prefer it. It will also not store as well as a traditional recipe but this has never been a problem for my family!

10 oz	plain flour	275 g
2-3 tsp	ground ginger	10-15 ml
1 tsp	bicarbonate of soda	5 ml
4 oz	soft margarine	100 g
2 oz	soft brown sugar	50 g
3 tbsp	black treacle	45 ml
½ pt	skimmed milk	275 ml
1	egg, beaten	1

Sieve together the flour, ginger and bicarbonate of soda. Add the remaining ingredients to the bowl and beat with a wooden spoon until thoroughly mixed. Pour into a lightly greased and base-lined 8-inch (20-cm) square shallow tin. Bake in a preheated oven at 150°C (300°F) Gas Mark 2 for 1 hour or until a skewer inserted comes out clean. Leave in the tin for a few minutes before turning out to cool completely on a wire rack. Cut into 16 squares.

PER SQUARE	
calories	130
g fat	6
g protein	3
g carbohydrate	17

Best eaten within 2-3 days.
Suitable for freezing.
Store in an airtight container.

Cherry and Walnut Loaf

When making cakes in which the fat and sugar are creamed together, you can usually reduce the amount of sugar by half as I have in this recipe.

4 oz	soft margarine	100 g
2 oz	caster sugar	50 g
1	egg, beaten	1
9 oz	self-raising flour	250 g
2 tsp	baking powder	10 ml
1 tsp	mixed spice	5 ml
	pinch of salt	
4 oz	chopped walnuts	100 g
4 oz	glacé cherries, rinsed, dried and chopped	100 g
7 oz	skimmed milk	200 ml

Cream the margarine and sugar together until pale and creamy. Gradually beat in the egg. Sift the flour, baking powder, spice and salt together. Stir in the walnuts and cherries. Fold the flour mixture and milk alternately into the creamed mixture to make a smooth batter. Pour the mixture into a lightly greased and base-lined 2 lb (900 g) loaf tin. Bake in a preheated oven at 180°C (350°F) Gas Mark 4 for 1-1¼ hours or until a skewer inserted comes out clean. Cool in the tin for 10 minutes before turning out on to a wire rack to cool completely. Cut into 12 slices.

PER SLICE	
calories	234
g fat	14
g protein	5
g carbohydrate	24

Best eaten within 1-2 days. Wrap well and store in an airtight container.

Cherry and Sultana Cake

This recipe makes a light fruit cake for a great teatime treat.

4 oz	glacé cherries, rinsed and dried	100 g
4 oz	sultanas	100 g
8 oz	self-raising flour	225 g
4 oz	soft margarine	100 g
2 oz	caster sugar	50 g
3	eggs, beaten	3
1	lemon, grated rind and juice	1
1 tsp	baking powder	5 ml
3 tbsp	skimmed milk	45 ml

Roughly chop the cherries and mix together with the sultanas and one third of the flour. Cream the margarine and sugar together until pale and creamy. Gradually add the eggs and remaining flour alternately, mixing well after each addition. Stir in the cherry mixture, lemon rind and juice, baking powder and milk. Spoon into a lightly greased and base-lined round 7-inch (18-cm) cake tin and level the top. Bake in a preheated oven at 180°C (350°F) Gas Mark 4 for 50-60 minutes or until a skewer inserted into the cake comes out clean. Allow to cool in the tin for 10 minutes before turning out on to a wire rack to cool completely. Cut into 12 slices.

PER SLICE	
calories	203
g fat	9
g protein	5
g carbohydrate	28

Best eaten within 2-3 days.

Shortbread

Shortbread is a traditional family favourite. However, as it is rather high in fat and calories, I would suggest including it in your diet as an occasional treat, rather than an everyday snack.

5 oz	soft margarine	150 g
4 oz	plain flour	100 g
3 oz	self-raising flour	75 g
1½ oz	caster sugar	40 g

Rub the margarine into the flours until the mixture resembles fine breadcrumbs. Stir in the sugar and knead together until a soft dough is formed, leaving the bowl clean. Press into an 8-inch (20-cm) tin and smooth the top. Flute the edges and prick all over with a fork. Mark into 8 portions. Bake in a preheated oven at 150°C (300°F) Gas Mark 2 for 50-60 minutes. Leave in the tin for 10 minutes before cooling completely on a wire rack. Sprinkle with a little granulated artificial sweetener if desired. Wrap in foil and store in an airtight container. Serves 8.

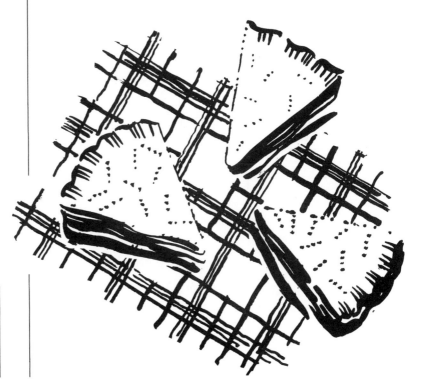

PER SERVING	
calories	230
g fat	16
g protein	2
g carbohydrate	21

Cheese and Bacon Loaf

A savoury bread which is delicious served warm.

4 oz	lean back bacon rashers	100 g
4 oz	plain flour	100 g
4 oz	plain wholemeal flour	100 g
1 tsp	bicarbonate of soda	5 ml
½ tsp	cream of tartar	2.5 ml
½ tsp	dried mustard powder	2.5 ml
2 oz	soft margarine	50 g
4 oz	cheddar, grated	100 g
5	spring onions, finely chopped	5
1	egg, beaten	1
¼ pt	semi-skimmed milk	150 ml

Grill the bacon until crisp. Drain on kitchen paper and cut into small pieces. Sift the flours, bicarbonate of soda, cream of tartar, and mustard powder into a bowl. Tip any bran remaining in the sieve back into the bowl. Rub in the margarine until the mixture resembles breadcrumbs. Stir in the bacon, 3 oz (75 g) of the cheese and the spring onions. Beat the egg and milk together and stir into the flour mixture. Mix well. Transfer to a lightly greased 2 lb (900 g) loaf tin and smooth the top. Sprinkle the remaining cheese over. Bake in a preheated oven at 200°C (400°F) Gas Mark 6 for 35-40 minutes or until a skewer when inserted comes out clean. Allow to cool in the tin for 5 minutes, before turning out on to a wire rack. Serve in slices, warm or cold. Cuts into approximately 10 slices.

PER SLICE	
calories	166
g fat	9
g protein	7
g carbohydrate	15

Best eaten the same day.
Suitable for freezing.

Wholemeal Bread

Easy-blend dried yeast should be stirred into the dry ingredients before adding the water unlike fresh or traditional dried yeast that needs to be added to liquid first.

2 lb	strong wholemeal flour	900 g
2 tsp	salt	10 ml
1	sachet easy-blend dried yeast	1
2 oz	soft margarine	50 g
1 pt	hand-hot water	550 ml

Place the flour, salt and yeast in a large bowl. Rub in the margarine and add enough water to make a soft dough.
Turn out on to a lightly floured board and knead for 10-15 minutes until smooth and elastic. Cover and leave to prove in a warm place until doubled in size (approximately 45 minutes). Re-knead the dough and divide equally to fit three 1 lb (450 g) greased loaf tins. Prove in a warm place until the dough is just above the top of the tins (approximately 60 minutes). Bake at 230°C (450°F) Gas Mark 8 for 30-40 minutes until browned. Cool on a wire rack. Makes three 1 lb (450 g) loaves. Each loaf cuts into approximately 16 slices.

PER 1 lb (450 g) LOAF	
calories	1053
g fat	20
g protein	38
g carbohydrate	191

If making 2 lb (900 g) loaves, these will require 30-40 minutes cooking time at the same temperature as for the smaller loaves.

Best eaten the same day. Suitable for freezing.

Granary Loaf

Home-made bread is delicious served warm: I find it easier to make using a table-top electric mixer with a dough hook.

2.2 lb	Granary flour	1 kg
2 tsp	salt	10 ml
1	sachet easy-blend dried yeast	1
3 tbsp	sunflower or corn oil	45 ml
1 pt	(approx) hand-hot water	550 ml
	a little beaten egg to glaze	

Mix the flour, salt and yeast together in a large bowl. Add the oil and water and mix well, adding a little extra water if necessary to make a pliable dough. Knead on a lightly floured surface until smooth and elastic. Divide the dough equally into 4 and shape to fit four 1 lb (450 g) greased loaf tins. Cover and prove for approximately 1 hour until the dough has rounded over the tops of the tins. Brush a little beaten egg on the tops and bake in a preheated oven at 230°C (450°F) Gas Mark 8 for 20-35 minutes until golden brown. Cool on a wire rack. Makes four 1 lb (450 g) loaves or two 2 lb (900 g) loaves.

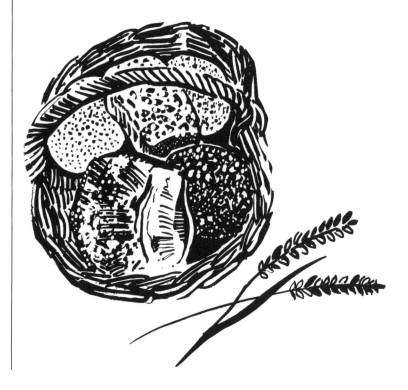

PER 1 lb (450 g) LOAF	
calories	926
g fat	13
g protein	32
g carbohydrate	175

Best eaten the same day.
Suitable for freezing.

Hot Cross Buns

8 oz	strong plain wholemeal flour	225 g
8 oz	strong plain flour	225 g
1 tsp	salt	5 ml
1 tsp	ground mixed spice	5 ml
1/2 tsp	ground cinnamon	2.5 ml
2 oz	soft margarine	50 g
1	sachet easy-blend dried yeast	1
1 oz	caster sugar	25 g
5 oz	currants	150 g
1/4 pt	warm skimmed milk	150 ml
1	egg, beaten	1
4 tbsp	(approx) warm water	60 ml
For the glaze		
1 tbsp	apricot jam	15 ml
3 tbsp	water	45 ml

Sift the flours, salt and spices into a large bowl, retaining the bran from the flour. Rub in the margarine. Stir in the yeast, sugar and currants. Make a well in the centre and add the milk, egg and enough water to form a soft dough. Turn out on to a lightly floured surface and knead until smooth and elastic. Alternatively, use a food processor or mixer. Place in an oiled bowl, cover with oiled plastic wrap and leave to rise in a warm place until doubled in size (approx 1-1 1/2 hours).

Knock back the dough and shape into 14 balls. Place well apart on lightly greased baking trays and flatten slightly. Cover with oiled plastic wrap and leave to prove for 30 minutes. Remove the plastic wrap and slash a cross in each bun. Bake in a preheated oven at 200°C (400°F) Gas Mark 6 for 15-20 minutes. Gently heat the jam and water together and use to brush over the buns whilst still hot. Cool on a wire rack. Makes 14.

PER BUN	
calories	174
g fat	4
g protein	5
g carbohydrate	31

Shortcrust Pastry

4 oz	plain flour	100 g
	pinch of salt	
2 oz	soft margarine	50 g
	cold water to mix	

PER QUANTITY OF PASTRY	
calories	640
g fat	37
g protein	3
g carbohydrate	67

Sieve the flour and salt into a bowl, tipping any bran in the sieve into the bowl. Rub in the margarine until the mixture resembles fine breadcrumbs. Add enough cold water to mix to a soft dough. Wrap in greaseproof paper and allow to chill for 30 minutes before rolling out. Use as required.

Desserts

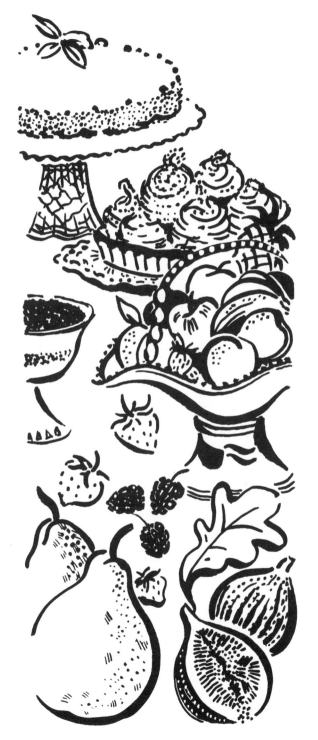

It's a myth that people with diabetes can't eat desserts containing sugar or indulgent puddings. With the following I've tried to cut down on fat or use less sugar where possible.

A truly old fashioned custard tart would have contained meat such as pigeons and other smaller birds for this was the Medieval version. What is in fact a much more modern recipe with sugar and spice is a nineteenth century development. We now consider this an old fashioned way of making custard thanks to (or because of) the invention of Alfred Bird who strove to find a substitute for custard because his wife was allergic to eggs.

Old Fashioned Baked Custard Tart

An old fashioned dessert which is delicious served chilled.

4 oz	plain flour	100 g
	a pinch of salt	
2 oz	soft margarine	50 g
1	egg yolk	1
3 tbsp	cold water	45 ml
1 oz	caster sugar	25 g
4	eggs, lightly beaten	4
12 fl oz	skimmed milk	350 ml
1 tsp	freshly grated nutmeg	5 ml

Sift the flour together with the salt. Rub in the margarine until the mixture resembles fine breadcrumbs. Stir in the egg yolk and enough cold water to form a soft dough. Wrap in greaseproof and chill for 15 minutes.

Roll out the pastry thinly on a lightly floured surface and use to line an 8-inch (20-cm) flan dish. Chill for 15-20 minutes. Bake blind in a preheated oven at 220°C (425°F) Gas Mark 7 for 5 minutes. Remove the paper and beans and cook for a further 5 minutes.

Meanwhile, lightly whisk the sugar and eggs together. Place the milk and half the nutmeg in a saucepan and warm gently. Pour on to the egg mixture. Strain the mixture into a jug and pour into the pastry case. Sprinkle with the remaining nutmeg.

Bake in a preheated oven at 220°C (425°F) Gas Mark 7 for 8 minutes. Reduce the temperature to 180°C (350°F) Gas Mark 4 and cook for a further 15-20 minutes or until the pastry is golden and the custard is just set.

Cool on a wire rack. Serve cold. Serves 8.

PER SERVING	
calories	163
g fat	9
g protein	7
g carbohydrate	14

Right:
Figs with Blackberry Sauce
(page 170)

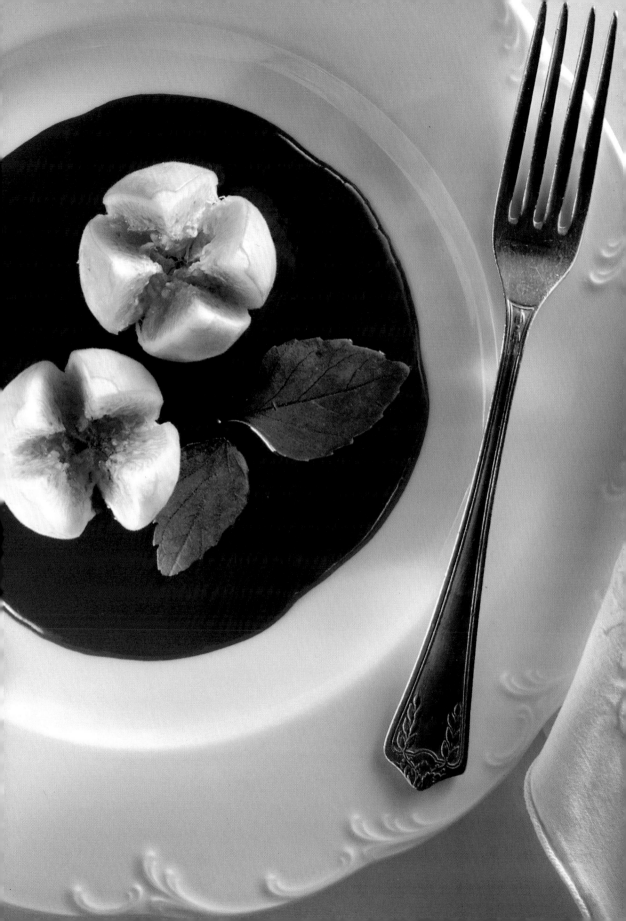

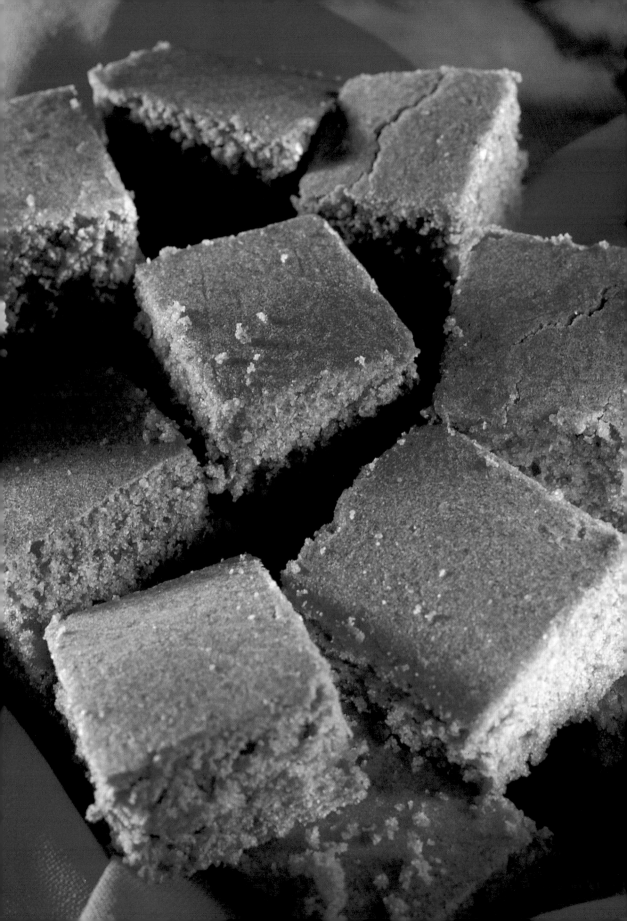

Apple Pie in a Walnut Pastry

The pastry has a lovely nutty flavour which complements the apple well. It is a fairly soft pastry and therefore needs to be chilled before rolling. Depending on your taste, you may prefer not to sweeten the apples or you could sprinkle a little extra sugar over the top of the pie after cooking.

For the pastry		
4 oz	plain flour	100 g
	a pinch of salt	—
2 oz	soft margarine	50 g
2 oz	walnuts, very finely chopped	50 g
For the filling		
2 lb	cooking apples	900 g
2-3 tbsp	caster sugar	30-45 ml
1/4 tsp	ground cinnamon	1.25 ml
	a little beaten egg to glaze	

To make the pastry, sift the flour into a bowl. Rub in the margarine until the mixture resembles fine breadcrumbs. Stir in the walnuts. Add enough cold water to form a soft dough. Wrap in greaseproof paper and chill in the refrigerator.

Meanwhile, peel, core and slice the apples and layer with the sugar, if using, to taste and spice in a 2-pt (1-litre) ovenproof pie dish. Roll out the pastry on a lightly floured board and cut a strip to cover the rim of the dish. Brush the rim with water and press the pastry down well to cover. Dampen the pastry edge with water and cover the dish with the pastry lid. Press down well and trim the edges. Reroll the trimmings and cut into leaves. Moisten with water and arrange on the pie. Glaze the pastry with a little beaten egg. Place the pie in a preheated oven at 220°C (425°F) Gas Mark 7 and cook for 25-30 minutes until golden. Cover with foil if the pastry is over-browning. Serve hot or cold. Serves 8.

PER SERVING	
calories	167
g fat	10
g protein	3
g carbohydrate	18

Left:
Quick Chocolate Squares
(page 129)

You can vary the fruit in an upside-down pudding to suit whatever is to hand. Peach slices or halves are a good choice. Try pear halves or stoned cherries; they are especially delicious with a little cocoa powder added to the sponge mixture.

Apricot Upside-Down Pudding

A variation on the traditional pineapple upside-down pudding. The sugar content has been reduced in this recipe by using fruit tinned in juice rather than syrup. I have also halved the amount of sugar in the sponge recipe compared with a traditional mixture.

1	can (14 oz/400 g) apricot halves in natural juice	1
6 tbsp	caster sugar	90 ml
6 oz	soft margarine	175 g
3	eggs, beaten	3
6 oz	self-raising flour	175 g
1 tsp	vanilla essence	5 ml
2 tbsp	hot water	30 ml

Drain the apricot halves, reserving the juice. Arrange the apricots flat side down in the bottom of a lightly greased and base-lined 8-inch (20-cm) round cake tin. Mix 4 tablespoons of the apricot juice with 2 tablespoons of sugar and spoon over the apricots. Cream the margarine and remaining sugar until pale and fluffy. Gradually beat in the eggs, beating well after each addition. Fold in the flour, vanilla essence and water. Spoon the mixture evenly into the cake tin and level the surface. Cook in a preheated oven at 180°C (350°F) Gas Mark 4 for 35-40 minutes until well risen, and a skewer when inserted comes out clean. Turn out on to a serving plate, remove the paper and serve warm with custard or half-fat cream. Serves 10.

PER SERVING	
calories	244
g fat	16
g protein	4
g carbohydrate	21

Put biscuits in a strong plastic bag and roll over with a rolling pin to crush them. If you buy a packet of biscuits and some are broken, crush them and store them in the freezer for instant use in desserts like this.

Cheat's Cheesecake

A simple dessert to make a mid-week meal seem special. It is very easy to make and takes very little preparation, yet looks impressive. Use chilled ingredients and serve as soon as possible otherwise the biscuits will lose their crunchiness.

6	digestive biscuits, crushed	6
5 oz	reduced-fat cream cheese	150 g
7 oz	plain virtually-fat-free fromage frais	200 g
1 tbsp	granulated artificial sweetener or caster sugar	15 ml
1/2 tsp	vanilla essence	2.5 ml
8 oz	raspberries, thawed if frozen	225 g
	a litte granulated sweetener or caster sugar to taste	

Divide the biscuits among 4 individual glass dishes. Beat the cream cheese, fromage frais, sweetener or sugar and vanilla essence together. Spoon on top of the crumbs. Divide the raspberries among the dishes, sprinkle with a little sweetener or sugar if desired. Serve immediately. Serves 4.

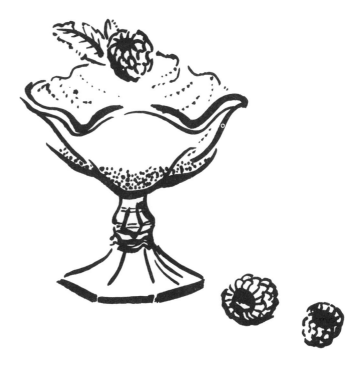

PER SERVING	
calories	217
g fat	13
g protein	6
g carbohydrate	19

Lemon and Sultana Cheesecake

This baked cheesecake has a lovely lemony flavour which complements the sultanas well.

5 oz	sultanas	150 g
3	lemons, finely grated rind and juice	3
5 oz	plain flour	150 g
5 oz	soft margarine	150 g
2-3 tbsp	water	30-45 ml
1 tbsp	cornflour	15 ml
14 oz	reduced-fat soft cheese	400 g
2-3 tbsp	caster sugar	30-45 ml
3	eggs, beaten	3
1 tsp	vanilla essence	5 ml

Place the sultanas, lemon rind and juice in a bowl and leave to soak for 30 minutes. Meanwhile, sift the flour into a bowl and rub in half the fat until the mixture resembles breadcrumbs. Stir in enough water to form a firm dough. Roll out on a lightly floured surface to line the base and sides of a 9-inch (23-cm) round, shallow loose-bottomed tin. Chill for 15 minutes. Bake the pastry blind in a preheated oven at 200°C (400°F) Gas Mark 6 for 10 minutes. Remove the paper and beans and cook for a further 5 minutes. Reduce the oven temperature to 160°C (325°F) Gas Mark 3.

Melt the remaining fat and beat in the cornflour, soft cheese, sugar, eggs, vanilla, sultanas and lemon juice. Beat well to mix thoroughly. Pour the mixture into pastry case and bake for 45 minutes at 160°C (325°F) Gas Mark 3 or until firm and golden. Allow to cool. Run a knife around the edge and remove from the tin. Chill before serving. Serves 10.

PER SERVING	
calories	323
g fat	24
g protein	5
g carbohydrate	23

Using Gelatine
Always add gelatine to liquid and not the other way round. When you are adding the dissolved gelatine to the mixture, there should not be a big temperature difference between the two. Never over heat gelatine; if it gets too hot it will not set.

Pineapple and Lemon Cheesecake

A light and refreshing cheesecake with a lovely pineapple flavour. Please note that the Department of Health still advise that pregnant women and the elderly should not eat raw eggs.

2 oz	soft margarine	50 g
6 oz	Hob Nob biscuits, finely crushed	175 g
1	can (8 oz/225 g) pineapple pieces in natural juice	1
1	packet ($\frac{1}{2}$ oz/11 g) gelatine	1
7 oz	reduced-fat soft cheese	200 g
1	carton (5 oz/150 g) low-fat natural yogurt	1
1	small lemon, grated rind and juice	1
3 tbsp	caster sugar	45 ml
2	egg whites	2

Melt the margarine and stir in the crushed biscuits until thoroughly mixed. Spread over the base of a 9-inch (23-cm) loose-bottomed tin. Chill in the refrigerator until required. Drain the pineapple and reserve the juice and 4 pieces.

Meanwhile, pour the reserved juice into a small bowl. Sprinkle the gelatine over the juice and leave to soften for 5 minutes. Stand the bowl over a pan of hot water and stir until the gelatine has dissolved. Set aside to cool slightly. Place the soft cheese, yogurt, lemon rind and juice in a food processor or liquidiser. Blend until smooth, then pour into a bowl. Add the pineapple to the processor and blend for a few seconds until finely chopped, but not a purée. Stir into the cheese mixture with the caster sugar to taste. Whisk the egg whites until stiff peaks form. Lightly fold the gelatine into the pineapple mixture and lastly fold in the egg whites. Pour the mixture over the biscuit crumb base and place in the refrigerator until set. Decorate with the reserved pineapple before serving. Serves 8.

PER SERVING	
calories	229
g fat	16
g protein	4
g carbohydrate	20

Mandarin Creams
When strawberries are not in season this makes an excellent storecupboard dessert.

Substitute an orange jelly and decorate with a well drained can of mandarin segments in natural juice.

Strawberry Creams

1	sachet sugar-free strawberry jelly	1
1/2 pt	boiling water	275 ml
1	can (14.5 oz/410 g) evaporated milk, chilled overnight	1

sliced fresh strawberries and mint sprigs, to decorate

Dissolve the jelly crystals in the boiling water. Set aside to cool for 5 minutes. Meanwhile, whisk the evaporated milk using an electric whisk or mixer until thickened and doubled in volume. Fold the jelly into the milk until thoroughly blended. Pour into four 1/2-pt (275-ml) jelly moulds or individual dishes. It won't all fit at first but as the jelly mixture settles, top up with the remaining mixture. Chill for approximately 3 hours, or until set. Dip the moulds in hot water for 10 seconds and gently turn out on to serving plates. Decorate with sliced fresh strawberries and mint sprigs. Serves 4.

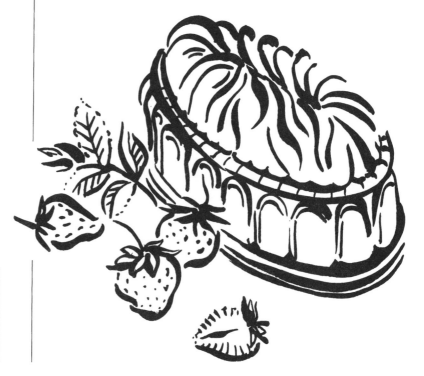

PER SERVING	
calories	170
g fat	9
g protein	9
g carbohydrate	15

Rhubarb and Ginger Fool

A simple dessert to make which has an unexpected 'kick' due to the ginger. It is also low in calories and fat.

1 lb	rhubarb, trimmed and cut into chunks	450 g
1 tbsp	finely grated root ginger	15 ml
3 tbsp	water	45 ml
2-3 tbsp	granulated artificial sweetener or caster sugar	30-45 ml

For the custard

1/2 pt	semi-skimmed milk	275 ml
2 tbsp	custard powder	30 ml
1 tbsp	granulated artificial sweetener or caster sugar	15 ml

Place the rhubarb, ginger and water into a saucepan. Cover and simmer for 5-10 minutes until soft. Cool. Reserve 4 pieces of rhubarb for decoration, stir the sweetener or sugar into the remainder. Make the custard with the milk and custard powder. Heat until very thick. Remove from the heat and stir in the sweetener or sugar. Fold the rhubarb into the custard and spoon into 4 individual glasses. Chill in the refrigerator. Decorate with the reserved rhubarb before serving. Serves 4.

PER SERVING	
calories	69
g fat	1
g protein	4
g carbohydrate	12

Tiramisu

This Italian dessert can be bought ready made at the shops but it can taste very synthetic. This recipe also has a lot fewer calories! Please note that the Department of Health currently advises that raw eggs should not be eaten by pregnant women or the elderly.

Tirami Su as the Italians would write it literally means 'pick me up'. If you like the creamy dessert but don't like coffee, make a chocolate version instead. Either use a chocolate liqueur or brandy and replace the strong coffee with a low-calorie chocolate drink such as Options.

1	egg, separated	1
2 tbsp	granulated artificial sweetener or caster sugar	30 ml
1/2 tsp	vanilla essence	2.5 ml
9 oz	reduced-fat cream cheese	250 g
1/4 pt	strong black coffee	150 ml
2 tbsp	coffee liqueur	30 ml
1/2	of one 7-inch (18-cm) cooked Victoria sandwich cake (see page 200 for recipe)	1/2
1/2 tsp	cocoa powder	2.5 ml

Place the egg yolk, sweetener, vanilla essence and cream cheese in a bowl and beat to a smooth consistency. Whisk the egg white until stiff and gently fold into the cream cheese mixture with a metal spoon. Mix the coffee and liqueur together in a bowl. Cut the sponge into strips and dip into the coffee and liqueur until it absorbs the mixture, but not until it falls apart.

Layer half the sponge in the base of 4 individual glass dishes, or 1 medium-sized serving dish, cutting into smaller pieces to fit if necessary. Cover with half the cheese mixture. Continue with another layer of sponge and finish with a layer of cheese mixture. Dust with cocoa powder and refrigerate for at least one hour until set. Serves 4.

PER SERVING	
calories	270
g fat	17
g protein	11
g carbohydrate	20

Pinolata

This is an Italian dessert cake which can be served with a fresh fruit salad.

2	eggs	2
2 oz	caster sugar	50 g
1	lemon, grated rind	1
4 oz	soft margarine	100 g
10 oz	self-raising flour	300 g
4 fl oz	dry sherry	160 ml
1 tsp	vanilla essence	5 ml
2 oz	pine nuts	50 g

Whisk the eggs and sugar together until pale and creamy. Beat in the lemon rind, margarine, flour, sherry and vanilla essence. Mix until well blended and smooth. Pour into a lightly greased and base-lined 9-inch (23-cm) deep cake tin. Sprinkle the pine nuts over the top. Bake in a preheated oven at 180°C (350°F) Gas Mark 4 for 30 minutes or until a skewer when inserted into the centre comes out clean. Serve warm. Cuts into 12.

PER SERVING	
calories	212
g fat	11
g protein	5
g carbohydrate	22

Best eaten the same day.

Banana Cream Pie

It will take around ten minutes to thicken the custard, so you will need some patience for this but it will thicken eventually. As the meringue is made with less sugar it will be slightly softer than an ordinary recipe, but is still just as nice.

1	quantity shortcrust pastry (see page 152)	1
2	eggs, separated	2
2 tbsp	cornflour	30 ml
1 tbsp	soft margarine	15 ml
1/2 pt	skimmed milk	275 ml
2 tbsp	granulated artificial sweetener or caster sugar (or to taste)	30 ml
1 tsp	vanilla essence	5 ml
2	medium bananas, sliced	2
3 tbsp	caster sugar	45 ml

Roll out the pastry on a lightly floured surface and use to line an 8-inch (20-cm) flan tin. Chill for 15 minutes in the refrigerator. Bake blind at 200°C (400°F) Gas Mark 6 for 10 minutes. Remove the baking beans and cook for a further 10 minutes until crisp.

Beat the egg yolks, cornflour and margarine in a heatproof bowl, until pale in colour. Bring the milk to the boil in a saucepan, then gradually whisk into the egg mixture. Cook the bowl of custard over a pan of simmering water, stirring constantly until thick. Remove from the heat and allow to cool slightly. Stir in the sweetener and vanilla essence.

Arrange the banana slices in the base of the pastry case, reserving a few for decoration (sprinkle these with a little lemon juice). Pour the custard over the banana slices. Whisk the egg whites until stiff, whisk in half the sugar, then fold in the rest. Pipe the meringue on top of the custard, leaving the centre uncovered. Bake at 150°C (300°F) Gas Mark 2 for 15-20 minutes until the meringue is golden. Arrange the remaining banana slices in the centre. Serve cold. Serves 8.

PER SERVING	
calories	194
g fat	7
g protein	5
g carbohydrate	29

Plum Sponge Pudding
Replace the apple and blackberries with 1½ lb (675 g) of ripe plums. Cut them in half and remove the stone before putting them in the dish. You probably will need very little if any sweetener.

Apple and Blackberry Sponge Pudding

I don't add sugar or a sweetener to fresh fruit when making pies or crumbles, or this dessert, as I find that the fruit is sweet enough. Using raspberries in place of the blackberries makes a nice variation.

1 lb	cooking apples, peeled, cored and sliced	450 g
8 oz	blackberries, washed	225 g
2 oz	caster sugar	50 g
2 oz	soft margarine	50 g
1 oz	self-raising wholemeal flour	25 g
½ tsp	baking powder	2.5 ml
1	lemon, grated rind and juice	1
1	size 2 egg, separated	1
4 fl oz	semi-skimmed milk	100 ml
1 oz	flaked almonds	25 g

Place the apples and blackberries in the base of a 2-pt (1-litre) ovenproof dish. Cream the sugar and margarine together until pale. Stir in the flour, baking powder, lemon rind and juice, egg yolk and milk and beat until smooth. (The mixture may look curdled.)

Whisk the egg white until stiff and fold into the mixture. Spoon over the apples and blackberries to cover. Sprinkle with the almonds. Place the dish in a roasting tin and fill with boiling water to halfway up the side of the dish.

Place in a preheated oven at 180°C (350°F) Gas Mark 4 and cook for 50 minutes until the sponge has risen and is golden. Serve hot. Serves 6.

PER SERVING	
calories	191
g fat	11
g protein	4
g carbohydrate	22

Pears with Raspberry Sauce

This dessert is made even more attractive if you choose nicely shaped and even-sized pears. Lay them sideways in the saucepan during cooking and turn occasionally so that they soak up the wine and are evenly coloured. Decorate the sauce with a little half-fat cream if desired.

4	medium pears	4
1/2 pt	red wine	275 ml
1-2	cinnamon sticks	1-2
4	cloves	4
1 tbsp	lemon juice	15 ml
For the sauce		
8 oz	raspberries, defrosted if frozen	225 g
2 tbsp	granulated artificial sweetener or caster sugar (or to taste)	30 ml

Peel the pears thinly, leaving the stalks intact. Remove the core with a knife or apple corer and cut a small piece from the base of each pear so they can stand up.

Place the pears in a medium-sized saucepan with the wine, cinnamon, cloves and lemon juice. Bring to the boil, cover and simmer for 15 minutes, basting and turning the pears occasionally. Remove from the heat and set aside.

To make the sauce, cook the raspberries for approximately 5 minutes over a gentle heat until the fruit is soft. Sieve the sauce to remove any pips. Stir in the sweetener to taste. Drain the pears and mix 5 tablespoons of the wine mixture with the raspberry sauce. Pour the sauce on to serving plates and add the pears. Decorate with fresh mint. Serves 4.

PER SERVING	
calories	125
g fat	0
g protein	2
g carbohydrate	18

The blackcurrants need to be very ripe for this dessert. If they seem to lack sweetness or flavour, simmer them in a tablespoon of water until their juice just starts to run. Cool completely before adding to the jelly.

If you can find some blueberries, these will make a delicious alternative to the blackcurrants.

Summer Fruit Layers

This dessert takes some time to prepare, but the result is impressive. Don't try to rush the jelly layers. Make sure that each layer is chilled until completely set. Keep the remaining jelly at room temperature until required. The carbohydrate per serving is negligible. To make frosted glasses, dip the rim of the glasses in a lemon half and then sugar.

1	sachet strawberry flavoured sugar-free jelly crystals	1
1/2 pt	boiling water	275 ml
1/2 pt	rosé wine	275 ml
4 oz	strawberries, hulled	100 g
4 oz	blackcurrants, de-strung	100 g
4 oz	raspberries	100 g
1/4 pt	whipping cream	150 ml

Place the jelly crystals into a jug with the boiling water and stir until dissolved. Allow to cool slightly, then stir in the wine. Leave until cool. Reserving 2 strawberries for decoration, thinly slice the remainder and place in the base of 8 small dessert glasses. Pour over a layer of jelly. Chill in the refrigerator until set. Repeat with a layer of blackcurrants and jelly and chill until set. Finally, repeat with a layer of raspberries and jelly. Chill until firm.

Whip the cream until stiff. Spoon a layer of cream on to the surface of each jelly. Place the remainder in a piping bag and pipe a swirl on to each dessert. Top with a slice of strawberry and serve chilled. Serve with thin wafer biscuits if desired. Serves 8.

PER SERVING	
calories	107
g fat	7
g protein	1
g carbohydrate	4

Autumn Fruits Steamed Pudding

Apples and blackberries are a classic combination and now that frozen fruits are widely available in the shops when out of season, you don't need to wait until Autumn to make this dessert. However, fruits are cheaper when in season, or better still, why not pick your own blackberries!

1	medium cooking apple, peeled, cored and sliced	1
2 tbsp	water	30 ml
8 oz	raspberries or blackberries, thawed if frozen	225 g
4 oz	soft margarine	100 g
2 oz	caster sugar	50 g
	a few drops of vanilla essence	
2	size 2 eggs, beaten	2
6 oz	self-raising flour	175 g
2 tbsp	hot water	30 ml

Cook the apple with water over a gentle heat until soft. Drain and arrange in the base of a lightly greased 2-pt (1-litre) pudding basin with the raspberries or blackberries. Cream the margarine and sugar together until pale. Add the vanilla essence and eggs a little at a time, beating well after each addition. Using a metal spoon, fold in the flours and water to give a dropping consistency. Spoon into the pudding basin to cover the fruit. Cover with greased greaseproof paper and foil and secure with string. Steam for 1½ hours. Serves 8.

PER SERVING	
calories	224
g fat	12
g protein	4
g carbohydrate	25

Peach and Raspberry Rice
Replace the apples and blackberries with fresh peaches and raspberries or for a winter treat use tinned peaches in natural juice and frozen raspberries and omit cooking the fruit.

Chilled Rice with Apple and Blackberry

Substitute fresh or frozen raspberries for the blackberries if they are not in season. If you use raspberries, you may not need as much sweetener, depending on your taste.

4 tbsp	pudding rice	60 ml
1 pt	skimmed milk	550 ml
1	lemon, finely grated rind and juice	1
1	vanilla pod, split open	1
3 tbsp	granulated artificial sweetener or caster sugar	45 ml
12 oz	eating apples, peeled, cored and sliced	350 g
8 oz	blackberries	225 g
1	carton (5 oz/150 g) low-fat natural yogurt	1

Place the rice, milk, lemon rind and vanilla pod in a medium-sized saucepan. Bring to the boil and simmer uncovered, stirring occasionally until the rice is tender and most of the milk is absorbed, approximately 30-40 minutes. Turn into a large bowl and stir in 1 tbsp (15 ml) of the sugar or sweetener. Leave to cool. Meanwhile, place the apples in a saucepan with 2 tbsp (30 ml) of the lemon juice. Cover tightly and simmer until the apples are just tender but still hold their shape. Add the blackberries and cook for just a few seconds. Pour the fruit into a bowl. Stir in the remaining sugar or sweetener, cool, cover and chill for 1 hour. Fold the yogurt into the rice, cover and chill for 1 hour.

To serve, layer the apple and rice mixture in 4 individual glasses, discarding the vanilla pod as you find it. Top each with a blackberry and a slice of apple. Serves 4.

PER SERVING	
calories	180
g fat	1
g protein	9
g carbohydrate	36

Pears with Ginger Sauce

A light, low-calorie dessert which provides a clean and refreshing end to a meal.

4	dessert pears, peeled, cored and thinly sliced	4
8 oz	virtually-fat-free fromage frais	225 g
1	small lemon, grated rind	1
2 tsp	granulated artificial sweetener or caster sugar	10 ml
2 tsp	finely grated fresh root ginger	10 ml
1 oz	pecan nuts, finely chopped	25 g

Arrange the pear slices on four serving plates. Mix together the fromage frais, lemon rind, sugar or sweetener and ginger. Arrange on the plates next to the pears, topped with the chopped nuts. Serve chilled. Serves 4.

PER SERVING	
calories	136
g fat	5
g protein	5
g carbohydrate	20

This tastes equally delicious with pear or a mixture of apple and pear.

Spiced Apple Pie in Filo Pastry

An apple pie which is low in fat and calories! Serve with a little half-fat cream or custard. Filo pastry is much lower in fat than ordinary shortcrust pastry, less than 2 g per 4 oz/100 g compared to around 30 g in the same weight of shortcrust pastry.

1 lb	cooking apples, peeled, cored and sliced	450 g
4 tbsp	water	60 ml
1/2 tsp	ground mixed spice	2.5 ml
1/2 tsp	ground cinnamon	2.5 ml
1 oz	sultanas	25 g
1 tbsp	caster sugar	15 ml
1	sheet filo pastry approx 18 x 11 inch (45 x 28 cm)	1
1/2 oz	soft margarine	15 g

Place the apples in a small saucepan with the water and spices. Cook over a gentle heat for 5 minutes. Stir in the sultanas and sweetener and spoon into a small, shallow ovenproof dish.

Brush one side of the filo pastry with the melted margarine and then tear it into pieces. Arrange the filo pastry over the apple with the 'buttered' side up. Bake in a preheated oven at 220°C (425°F) Gas Mark 7 for 15 minutes, or until the pie is golden brown. Serve warm with half-fat cream. Serves 4.

PER SERVING	
calories	94
g fat	4
g protein	1
g carbohydrate	15

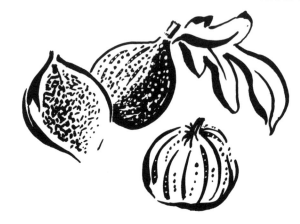

Figs with Blackberry Sauce

Depending on the sweetness of the blackberries, you may not need to add any sweetener, or just a little to take away any sharpness from the fruit.

8	ripe fresh figs	8
8 oz	blackberries	225 g
1 tsp	arrowroot	5 ml
1-2 tsp	granulated artificial sweetener or caster sugar (or to taste)	5-10 ml

A perfect fig will be unblemished and will just yield when you hold it without pressing on it. It can be any colour from pale green to deep purple.

Cut the stalks off the figs. Make two cuts in each fig in a cross shape, from the stalk end, three-quarters of the way through. Open up to resemble flowers. Place two figs on each of four serving plates. Place the blackberries and 2 tbsp (30 ml) of water in a small saucepan. Cook for 2-3 minutes until soft. Mix the arrowroot to a smooth paste with 2 tsp (10 ml) of water. Stir in the blackberry mixture and boil for 1 minute to thicken.

Push the blackberries through a sieve to remove the pips. Stir in the sugar or sweetener to taste. Pour a little blackberry sauce over each fig. Serve the remaining sauce separately in a jug. Serves 4.

PER SERVING	
calories	99
g fat	1
g protein	2
g carbohydrate	23

Chilled Lemon Soufflé

I remember making my first lemon soufflé during my 'A' level Home Economics class. This recipe uses a granulated sweetener to reduce the sugar content and also the calories. It makes a refreshing dessert to end a dinner party.

3	lemons, grated rind and juice	3
6	eggs, size 2, separated	6
5 tbsp	caster sugar	75 ml
2 tbsp	powdered gelatine	30 ml
3/4 pt	whipping cream	425 ml
2 oz	chopped mixed nuts, toasted	50 g
	blanched shreds of lemon rind to decorate	

Tie a double strip of greaseproof paper around a 1½-pt (900-ml) soufflé dish to make a 3-inch (7.5-cm) collar. Lightly brush the inside of the paper with a little oil.

With an electric whisk, whisk the lemon rind, egg yolks and sugar together in a bowl until pale. Pour 7 tablespoons (105 ml) of the lemon juice into a small bowl, sprinkle in the gelatine and leave to soak for 2-3 minutes. Place the bowl over a pan of simmering water until the gelatine dissolves. Allow to cool slightly, then stir into the egg yolk mixture.

Lightly whip the cream until it forms peaks and is suitable for piping. Reserving a little for piping, fold the remainder into the egg yolk mixture.

Whisk the egg whites in a large bowl until they form stiff peaks. With a large metal spoon, carefully fold into the egg yolk mixture. Gently pour the mixture into the prepared soufflé dish. Chill for at least 4 hours until set.

Carefully ease the paper collar away from the soufflé with a knife dipped in hot water. Press the toasted nuts around the edge of the soufflé with a palette knife. Decorate the top with cream whirls and the blanched shreds of lemon rind. Serve as soon as possible. Serves 6.

PER SERVING	
calories	409
g fat	40
g protein	10
g carbohydrate	3

Custard

You can easily reduce the sugar content of desserts by making your custard with an artificial sweetener. I use a granulated sweetener which can be used spoon for spoon in place of sugar. Sweeteners should generally be added after the custard is boiled as some types lose their sweetness at high temperatures.

2 tbsp	custard powder	30 ml
1/2 pt	skimmed milk or semi-skimmed	275 ml
	caster sugar or artificial sweetener (to taste)	

PER 1/2 pt (275 ml)	
calories	233
g fat	5
g protein	10
g carbohydrate	41

   Blend the custard powder with 2 tablespoons (30 ml) of the milk. Warm the remainder of the milk in a saucepan. Whisk in the custard powder mixture until thoroughly mixed and continue heating and whisking until thick and creamy. Remove from the heat and add the sugar or sweetener to taste. Makes 1/2 pt (275 ml).

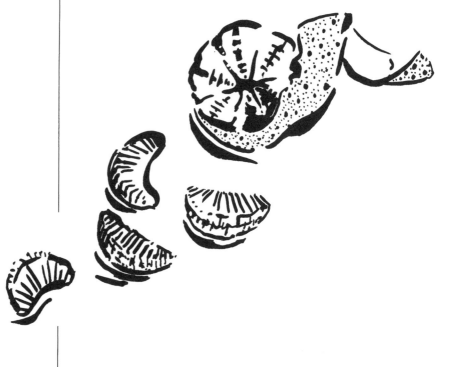

Spiced Mandarin Gateau

This elegant dessert is perfect for entertaining and would be ideal at Christmas for those who prefer a lighter dessert than Christmas pudding.

4	size 2 eggs	4
3 oz	caster sugar	75 g
4 oz	plain flour	100 g
1/4 tsp	ground ginger	1.25 ml
1/4 tsp	mixed spice	1.25 ml
1 oz	soft margarine, melted and cooled	25 g
2 tsp	caster sugar	10 ml

For the filling

1/2 pt	whipping cream	275 ml
2 tbsp	granulated artificial sweetener or caster sugar	30 ml
1	can (11 oz/300 g) mandarin segments in natural juice, drained	1

Lightly grease and base-line a 12 x 10-inch (30 x 25-cm) Swiss roll tin. Lightly dredge with a little plain flour.

Place the eggs and sugar in the bowl of an electric mixer and whisk on maximum speed until the mixture is thick and the whisk leaves a trail when lifted. (Alternatively, whisk in a bowl over a saucepan of gently simmering water.)

Sift the flour and spices together twice, and fold lightly and evenly into the egg mixture. Finally, fold in the cooled margarine using a large spoon. Pour the mixture into the prepared tin and level the surface. Bake in a preheated oven at 190°C (375°F) Gas Mark 5 for 15-20 minutes, or until pale brown and springy to the touch.

Have ready a sheet of baking parchment, sprinkled with the two teaspoons of sugar. Turn the sponge out on to the paper and peel off the lining paper immediately. Trim the edges of the sponge with a sharp knife. Roll up from the short edge whilst still warm, with the paper inside.

Leave to cool completely on a wire rack. Whip the cream until stiff and lightly fold in the sugar or sweetener to taste. Unroll the sponge and remove the paper. Spread three-quarters of the cream over the sponge. Reserving 8 of the mandarins for decoration, arrange the remainder over the cream, re-roll the sponge and carefully place on a serving dish.

Pipe the reserved cream down the centre of the roll and decorate with the remaining mandarins. Chill in the refrigerator until ready to serve. Serves 10.

PER SERVING	
calories	234
g fat	16
g protein	5
g carbohydrate	20

Note: due to the reduced sugar content, the meringue topping will have a slightly soft texture.

Lemon and Lime Meringue Pie

A variation of a family favourite.

For the pastry

4 oz	plain flour	100 g
1 oz	soft margarine	25 g
1 oz	white vegetable fat (such as Flora)	25 g
2-3 tbsp	water	30-45 ml

For the filling

1	small lemon, finely grated rind and juice	1
1	small lime, finely grated rind and juice	1
1 oz	soft margarine	25 g
3 tbsp	cornflour	45 ml
2	size 3 egg yolks	2
1 tbsp	caster sugar (or to taste)	15 ml

For the meringue

2	egg whites	2
2 tbsp	caster sugar	30 ml

Sieve the flour into a bowl. Rub in the margarines until the mixture resembles fine breadcrumbs. Add enough cold water to bind and knead to a soft dough.

Roll out the pastry on a lightly floured surface and use to line an 8-inch (20-cm) flan dish. Chill for 15 minutes.

Bake the pastry blind in a preheated oven at 200°C (400°F) Gas Mark 6 for 10 minutes. Remove the paper and baking beans and cook for a further 5 minutes. Reduce the oven temperature to 150°C (300°F) Gas Mark 2.

Meanwhile, prepare the filling. Make up the lemon and lime juice to ½ pint (275 ml) with cold water and place in a saucepan with the rind of the lemon and lime, margarine and cornflour. Bring to the boil and cook for 2-3 minutes, whisking continuously, until thickened and smooth. Allow to cool slightly, then beat in the egg yolks and the sweetener to taste. Pour into the flan case.

Whisk the egg whites until stiff peaks form. Carefully fold in the sugar and pile on to the flan case to cover the filling completely.

Bake the pie in the preheated oven for 20-25 minutes until golden brown. Serve hot or cold. Serves 8.

PER SERVING	
calories	165
g fat	9
g protein	3
g carbohydrate	20

Nectarine and Raspberry Fool

A virtually-fat-free dessert using fresh summer fruits. For a special finish, dip the rim of the sundae glasses in a fresh lemon half and then coat with artificial sweetener before filling with the fool mixture.

2	ripe nectarines	2
5 oz	raspberries, fresh or frozen	150 g
12 oz	virtually-fat-free fromage frais	350 g
1	carton (5 oz/150 g) low-fat natural yogurt	1
3 tbsp	granulated artificial sweetener or caster sugar (or to taste)	45 ml
	mint leaves to decorate	

Halve and stone the nectarines. Place in a blender or food processor and purée until smooth. Add a little sugar or sweetener to taste and set side. Reserving four for decoration, purée the remaining raspberries until smooth and strain through a sieve if desired to remove the pips. Pour into the base of four sundae dishes. Lightly fold the fromage frais and yogurt together, and add a little sugar or sweetener to taste.

Layer the yogurt mixture and nectarine purée in the sundae dishes, finishing with a layer of yogurt. Chill before serving, decorated with the reserved raspberries and mint leaves. Serves 4.

PER SERVING	
calories	108
g fat	1
g protein	10
g carbohydrate	17

Frozen Orange Cups

I find it easier to scoop out the flesh using a sharp knife to score around the outside and a spoon to scoop it out. This is a very refreshing dessert and is particularly suitable for serving in the summer months.

4	large oranges	4
2	cartons (5 oz/150 g) low-fat natural yogurt	2
7 oz	reduced-fat soft cream cheese	200 g
4 tbsp	granulated artificial sweetener or caster sugar	60 ml
	sprigs of fresh mint to decorate	

PER SERVING	
calories	200
g fat	12
g protein	6
g carbohydrate	16

Trim a small amount from the base of each orange so that they stand upright. Cut away the tops and set aside. Scoop out the orange flesh and place in a food processor or liquidiser with the yogurt and cream cheese. Add the sugar or sweetener and process for 10-20 seconds, or until smooth. Pass through a sieve if desired. Pour into a freezerproof container. Freeze the orange cups and the ice cream for 4 hours, mashing the ice cream with a fork after 2 hours to get rid of ice crystals. (Alternatively, you can process the mixture in the food processor or liquidiser.) Remove the ice cream from the freezer 10 minutes before serving. Serve in scoops in the orange cups. Decorate with mint. Serves 4.

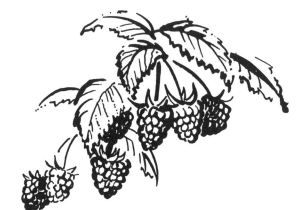

Raspberry Ice

Freeze this mixture in ice lolly moulds for great sugar-free treats for children and adults alike.

An economical dessert to make. Vary the flavour by using other soft fruits such as strawberries or blackcurrants.

1	can (14 oz/400 g) evaporated milk chilled overnight	1
12 oz	fresh raspberries	350 g

Whisk the evaporated milk using an electric food mixer until thick and creamy and doubled in volume. Purée the raspberries using a liquidiser or food blender and sieve to remove the pips. Whisk into the evaporated milk until evenly mixed. Turn into a rigid freezerproof container. Cover and freeze for 1 hour or until starting to freeze around the edges. Whisk well, then re-freeze until firm. Remove from the freezer and place in the refrigerator 30 minutes before serving to soften. Serve in scoops with fresh fruit. Serves 8.

PER SERVING	
calories	86
g fat	5
g protein	5
g carbohydrate	6

Summer Fruit Crumble

A dessert which can be enjoyed all year round. I've not added any extra sugar.

2	packets (1 lb/450 g) frozen mixed summer fruits	2
2 oz	soft margarine	50 g
3 oz	porridge oats	75 g
3 oz	no-added-sugar muesli	75 g

Place the summer fruits in a saucepan and heat gently until the juices begin to run and the fruit softens. Transfer to an ovenproof dish. To prepare the crumble, rub the margarine spread into the porridge oats until they have blended well, then mix with the muesli. Scatter the crumble over the fruit and cook at 190°C (375°F) Gas Mark 5 for 25 minutes. Serve hot with a little half-fat cream or custard. Serves 8.

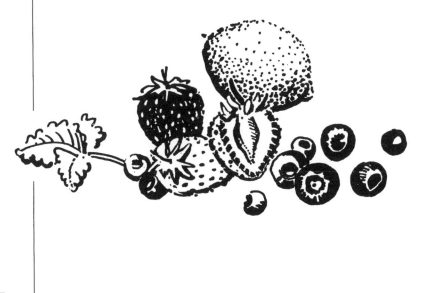

PER SERVING	
calories	144
g fat	7
g protein	4
g carbohydrate	18

Lime Torte

I have to thank our friends Jo and Howard for the origin of this recipe. Jo made a dessert from a supermarket recipe card which used mascarpone cheese and I thought it must be possible to use a lower-fat cheese and to reduce the sugar content. It is still, however, quite high in calories and would be suitable for entertaining rather than an everyday dessert.

6 oz	Hob Nob biscuits, crushed	175 g
2 oz	soft margarine	50 g
2	cartons (7 oz/200 g) reduced-fat soft cheese	2
3 tbsp	caster sugar	45 ml
2	limes, finely grated rind and juice	2
To decorate		
1	lime, shredded rind	1

Mix together the crushed biscuits and melted fat and press into the base of a 7-inch (18-cm) loose-bottomed cake tin.

Place the soft cheese, sugar, finely grated lime rind and juice in a bowl and beat together. Spread over the biscuit base. Chill for at least 2 hours. Decorate with shreds of lime rind before serving. Serves 6.

PER SERVING	
calories	345
g fat	29
g protein	3
g carbohydrate	20

Chocolate and Strawberry Roulade

3	size 2 eggs	3
3 oz	caster sugar	75 g
4 oz	self-raising flour	100 g
1/2 oz	cocoa powder	15 g
1 tbsp	warm water	15 ml
1 tsp	caster sugar	5 ml
9 oz	virtually-fat-free fromage frais	250 g
2-3 tbsp	granulated artificial sweetener or caster sugar (or to taste)	30-45 ml
8 oz	fresh strawberries, hulled and sliced	225 g

Whisk the eggs and sugar together using an electric food mixer for 5 minutes, or until pale and thick and the whisk leaves a trail in the mixture for a few seconds when lifted.

Sift the flour and cocoa together, tip any bran remaining in the sieve into the bowl. Fold in carefully with the water using a figure of eight movement. Pour the mixture into a lightly greased and lined 13 x 9-inch (32.5 x 23-cm) Swiss roll tin, tapping the mixture into the corners of the tin to cover the surface evenly. Bake in a preheated oven at 220°C (425°F) Gas Mark 7 for 8-10 minutes or until well risen and the cake springs back when lightly touched with a finger tip.

Turn on to a clean sheet of non-stick baking paper sprinkled with 1 teaspoon of caster sugar, and remove the lining paper. Trim the edges of the cake very thinly and roll up with the clean paper inside. Cool completely on a wire rack.

Lightly mix the fromage frais and sugar or sweetener together. Unroll the sponge carefully and spread with fromage frais. Scatter the strawberries over and roll up carefully. Sprinkle a little sweetener over the top if liked. Serve sliced. For a special occasion, whip 1/4 pt (150 ml) of whipping cream to fill the roulade. Serves 10.

PER SERVING	
calories	117
g fat	3
g protein	5
g carbohydrate	20

This dish is super made with stoned plums or ready-to-eat prunes in place of the cherries.

Clafouti

Clafouti is a French dessert recipe which I've adapted here to reduce the sugar and fat content. I make this recipe when cherries are in season otherwise the dish can prove to be rather expensive.

3 tbsp	plain flour	45 ml
	a pinch of salt	
3	eggs, beaten	3
4 tbsp	caster sugar	60 ml
3/4 pt	semi-skimmed milk	425 ml
12 oz	fresh red cherries, stoned	350 g
1/2 oz	soft margarine	15 g

Sift together the flour and salt into a bowl, then beat in the eggs and sugar. Heat the milk until almost boiling and beat into the egg mixture.

Lightly grease a large, shallow ovenproof dish and arrange the cherries over the base. Pour the batter over the top and dot with the margarine.

Bake in a preheated oven at 220°C (425°F) Gas Mark 7 for approximately 20-25 minutes until the custard is set and golden brown. Serves 8.

PER SERVING	
calories	126
g fat	5
g protein	5
g carbohydrate	16

Children's Recipes

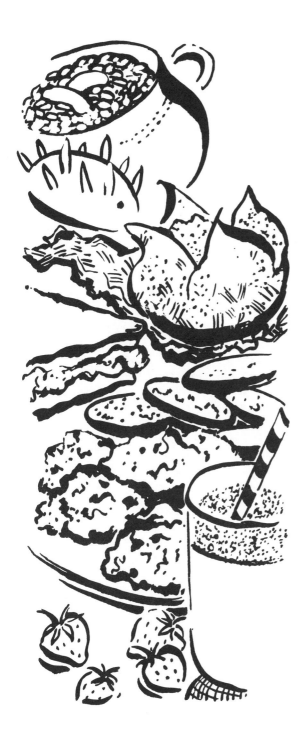

I had a lot of fun trying out these recipes and hearing the comments from my nieces Katie and Amy and cousin Emma. Unfortunately, my daughter Jade was too young at the time to join in! Many of the recipes are simple enough for children to make themselves, (with a helping hand here and there) but don't forget to make clearing up the mess part of the fun of cooking!

Chicken Wait-and-See Bake

When we asked my Mum what was for dinner when we were younger, she often replied 'Wait and see!'. This is a useful dish to serve on a Monday as you can use any cooked chicken left over from a Sunday roast for this recipe. Vary the vegetables to suit your children's tastes. For example, peas could be used instead of sweetcorn, and carrots in place of the broccoli.

1½ oz	soft margarine	40 g
1	medium onion, finely chopped	1
2 tbsp	plain flour	30 ml
¾ pt	semi-skimmed milk	425 ml
12 oz	broccoli spears, lightly cooked and drained	350 g
4 oz	drained weight canned sweetcorn	100 g
8 oz	cooked chicken, diced	225 g
	salt and freshly ground black pepper	
2 oz	cheddar, grated	50 g

Melt the margarine in a medium-sized saucepan and cook the onion over a gentle heat for 5 minutes until soft. Stir in the flour and cook for 1 minute. Gradually blend in the milk and bring to the boil, stirring constantly. Cook for 1-2 minutes, until thick. Stir in the broccoli, sweetcorn and cooked chicken and season to taste.

Turn the mixture into an ovenproof dish and sprinkle with the cheese. Bake in a preheated oven at 180°C (350°F) Gas Mark 4 for 25 minutes until golden brown. Serve with jacket potatoes and freshly cooked vegetables. Serve hot. Serves 4.

PER SERVING	
calories	324
g fat	17
g protein	24
g carbohydrate	20

It is much easier to persuade children to eat what is good for them if it is fun. Serve the Cowboy's Supper in true western style on enamel camping plates and let them sit in the garden or for a winter treat make a tent from an old blanket and the clothes horse.

Cowboy's Supper

This is a quick and easy family supper which is convenient to make if you don't need to have the oven on for anything else, since it is just cooked on the hob. Sausages and beans are a traditional combination which is popular with children. Serve with mashed potato for a campfire supper.

1 lb	sausages	450 g
1 tbsp	olive or corn oil	15 ml
1	large onion, sliced	1
2	large carrots, diced	2
1	can (14 oz/400 g) chopped tomatoes	1
1 tbsp	dried mixed herbs	15 ml
1	can (8 oz/225 g) baked beans	1
1/4 pt	hot vegetable or chicken stock	150 ml
	salt and freshly ground black pepper	

Grill the sausages under a hot grill until browned and cooked through. Cut into bite-sized pieces and set aside.

Heat the oil in a large saucepan and cook the onion and carrots for 5 minutes, stirring occasionally. Stir in the sausages and the remaining ingredients. Bring to the boil, cover and simmer for 20-25 minutes or until the sauce has thickened slightly and the vegetables are tender.

Serve with mashed potatoes or pasta. Serves 4.

PER SERVING	
calories	555
g fat	40
g protein	17
g carbohydrate	32

Vegetable Thatch Pie
Replace some of the potato
with carrots and parsnips for a
tasty topping. Just boil them
and mash them altogether.

Cheesy Shepherd's Pie

If you use a non-stick pan to cook mince, you don't need to add
any oil as it will cook in its own fat. Even with lean mince you
can still pour off a lot of excess fat when it is cooked. My niece
Amy (7) commented 'I like the brown stuff and I like the white
stuff, yes it's nice, lovely'. Her sister Katie and cousin Emma
both agreed it was nice.

2 lb	lean minced beef	900 g
1	large onion, finely chopped	1
2 tbsp	tomato purée	30 ml
1	can (14 oz/400 g) tomatoes	1
1/2 pt	beef stock	275 ml
	salt and freshly ground black pepper	
2 lb	potatoes, peeled and halved	900 g
4 tbsp	skimmed milk	60 ml
1/2 oz	soft margarine	15 g
4 oz	frozen peas	100 g
1 oz	cheddar, grated	25 g

Cook the mince and onion in a non-stick pan for 5 minutes
until browned. Drain off the excess fat. Stir in the tomato purée,
tomatoes and stock. Season to taste. Bring to the boil, cover and
simmer for 45 minutes.

Meanwhile, boil the potatoes in lightly salted water for
20-25 minutes until cooked. Drain and mash together with the
milk and margarine. Season to taste. Stir the peas into the
mince mixture. Spoon into a 21/2-pt (1.2-litre) ovenproof dish.
Cover with the mashed potato. Sprinkle with the grated cheese.
Place in a preheated oven at 180°C (350°F) Gas Mark 4 for
25 minutes until golden. Serves 6.

PER SERVING	
calories	432
g fat	13
g protein	50
g carbohydrate	31

Bacon and Cheese Stuffed Baked Potatoes

Baked potatoes are a firm family favourite and very easy to make. Vary the fillings by using lean ham, tuna, or perhaps cooked mushrooms, for a vegetarian option, in place of the bacon.

4	baking potatoes, approximately 6 oz (175 g) each, scrubbed	4
4 oz	lean back bacon rashers	100 g
2 tbsp	chopped fresh parsley	30 ml
4 oz	double Gloucester cheese, grated	100 g
1 tbsp	tomato purée	15 ml
	salt and freshly ground black pepper	

Prick the potatoes and bake at 180°C (350°F) Gas Mark 4 for approximately 1 hour until cooked. Meanwhile, grill the bacon until cooked. Drain on kitchen paper and chop.

Cut the cooked potatoes in half lengthways. Leave until cool enough to handle, then carefully scoop out the flesh, leaving the skins intact.

Mash the potato flesh and mix with the bacon, parsley, cheese and tomato purée. Season to taste. Spoon the mixture back into the reserved skins. Return to the oven and cook for a further 15 minutes to heat through. Serves 4.

PER SERVING	
calories	271
g fat	11
g protein	15
g carbohydrate	30

Crispy Scotch Eggs

Children will enjoy helping you to shape the sausagemeat around the eggs. The coating of the Scotch Eggs comes out very crisp from baking them in the oven and this way is a lot more healthy than the traditional fried method.

4	hard-boiled eggs, shelled	4
2 tsp	plain flour	10 ml
1 lb	sausagemeat	450 g
½	egg, beaten	½
3 oz	stale (wholemeal) breadcrumbs	75 g

Roll the eggs in the flour. Divide the sausagemeat into four even portions. Flatten the sausagemeat out and place an egg in the middle. With wetted hands, mould the sausagemeat around the egg. Dip each coated egg into the beaten egg and then roll in the breadcrumbs. Place on a baking tray and cook in a preheated oven at 190°C (375°F) Gas Mark 5 for 25-30 minutes until brown and crisp.

When cool, dip a sharp knife in water and halve each Scotch Egg. Chill in the refrigerator until required. Makes 8 halves.

PER SERVING	
calories	272
g fat	21
g protein	10
g carbohydrate	11

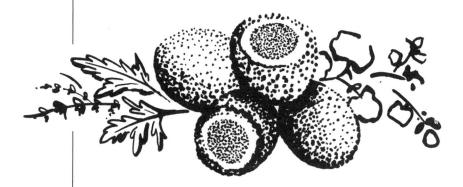

Family Favourite Bolognese Sauce

Spaghetti Bolognese is a favourite with young children and is very enjoyable to eat, even if it can be a bit messy! Adding extra vegetables such as carrots and mushrooms makes the meat go further and I think adds extra interest to this recipe. My friend's little girl, Coral, delights in recognising the mushrooms as she finds them.

Right:
Beany Burgers (page 188) and Strawberry Milkshake (page 195)

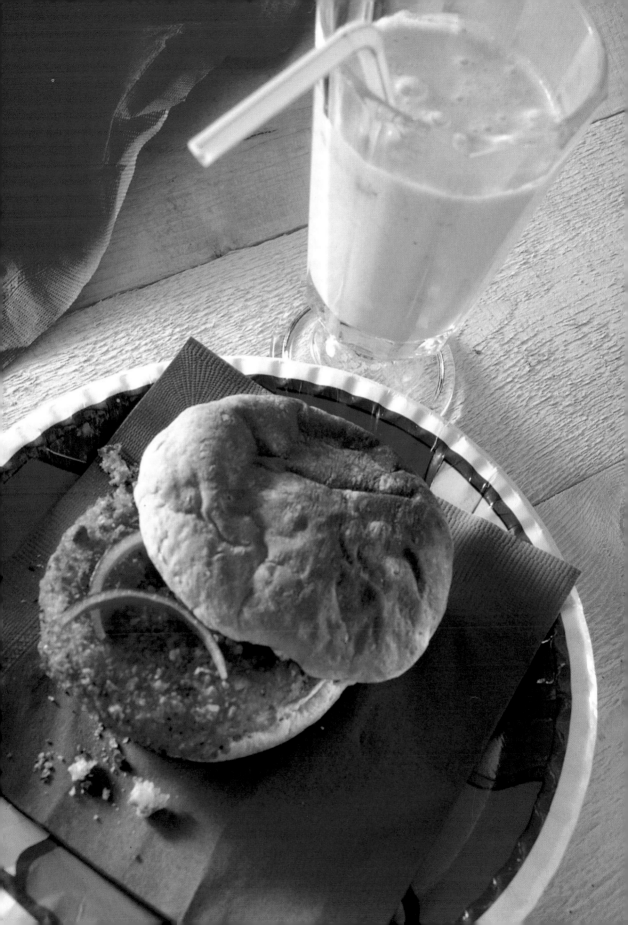

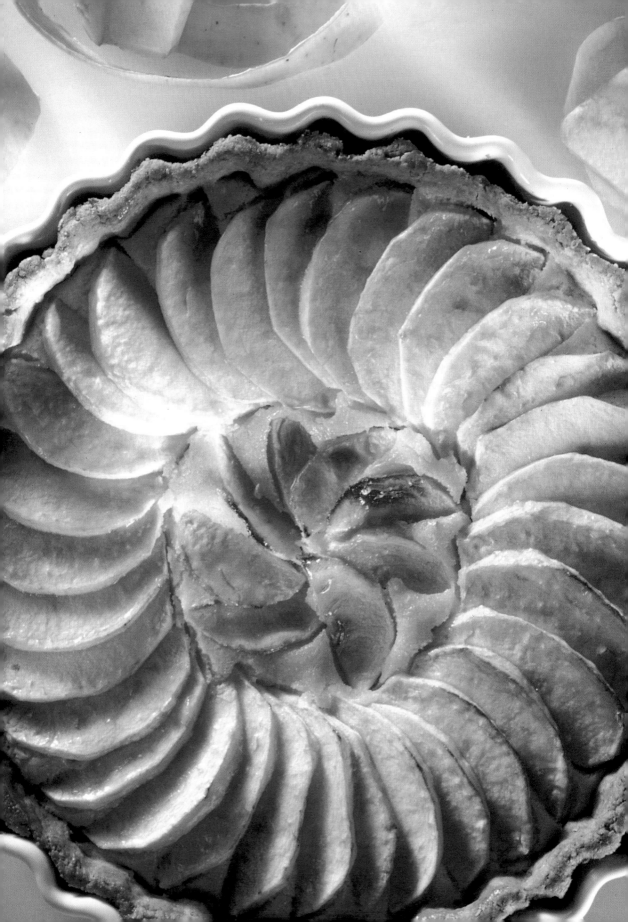

1 lb	lean minced beef	450 g
1	medium onion, finely chopped	1
1	clove garlic, crushed (optional)	1
2	large carrots, finely diced	2
8 oz	mushrooms, sliced	225 g
1	can (14 oz/400 g) chopped tomatoes	1
2 tbsp	tomato purée	30 ml
1/2 pt	beef stock, boiling	275 ml
1/2 tsp	dried oregano	2.5 ml
1/2 tsp	dried basil	2.5 ml
	salt and freshly ground black pepper	

Place the minced beef, onion and garlic if using, in a large nonstick pan and fry until browned, stirring constantly. Drain off any excess fat. Add the remaining ingredients and season to taste. Stir well. Bring to the boil, lower the heat and simmer for 40 minutes, stirring occasionally. Serve immediately with freshly cooked spaghetti. Serves 4-5.

PER SERVING	
calories	235
g fat	7
g protein	35
g carbohydrate	9

Crispy Baked Coley

A simple dish which is quick to prepare and to cook; ideal for a weekday meal. Serve with boiled new potatoes, or pasta and freshly cooked vegetables.

4	coley fillets (6 oz/175 g), skinned	4
4	slices lean ham	4
2-3 tbsp	lemon juice	30-45 ml
	salt and freshly ground black pepper	
1 oz	cheddar, grated	25 g
1 oz	fresh breadcrumbs	25 g

Lay the fillets skinned side uppermost on a board. Top each fillet with a slice of ham and sprinkle with a little lemon juice and seasoning.

Roll up the fillets from head to tail and place in an ovenproof dish. Secure with a cocktail stick if necessary. Cover and bake in a preheated oven at 190°C (375°F) Gas Mark 5 for 25-30 minutes.

PER SERVING	
calories	196
g fat	4
g protein	36
g carbohydrate	4

Left:
Normandy Apple Flan
(page 204)

Mix the cheese and breadcrumbs together. Remove the cover from the fish and spoon the cheese mixture over the top. Return to the oven for a further 5 minutes until the topping is crisp and golden brown. Serves 4.

Beany Burgers

I use a dried bean mixture, available prepacked in my local supermarket. Remember that the beans will need soaking overnight before cooking.

6 oz	dried mixed beans, such as chick peas, kidney beans, pinto beans, soaked overnight	175 g
1 tbsp	olive or sunflower oil	15 ml
1	small onion, finely chopped	1
1	large carrot, grated	1
1 tsp	yeast extract	5 ml
1 tsp	dried mixed herbs	5 ml
1 oz	fresh breadcrumbs	25 g
	salt and freshly ground black pepper	
	a little oil for brushing	

Drain the soaked beans and rinse thoroughly. Place in a large saucepan and cover with cold water. Bring to the boil and boil vigorously for 10 minutes. Reduce the heat and simmer for 1 hour until the beans are soft. Drain well.

Meanwhile, heat the oil in a small pan and cook the onions over a moderate heat until soft. Drain thoroughly on kitchen paper.

Place the beans with the onions and the remaining ingredients in a food processor or liquidiser and process until almost smooth. Season to taste.

Using wetted hands, shape the mixture into 6 burgers. Chill for at least 30 minutes.

Brush the burgers with a little oil and grill under a hot grill for approximately 15 minutes, turning once. Serve hot in toasted wholemeal baps. Serves 6.

It is best to cook pulses in unsalted water until they are almost tender as salt tends to toughen them, particularly with peas and beans. Add any salt about 15 minutes before the end of the cooking time.

PER SERVING	
calories	131
g fat	3
g protein	7
g carbohydrate	20

Baked Bean Lasagne

A good vegetarian option if you use a vegetarian cheese.

1 tbsp	olive or sunflower oil	15 ml
1	large onion, finely chopped	1
5 oz	mushrooms, sliced	150 g
1	can (15 oz/425 g) baked beans	1
1 tbsp	tomato purée	15 ml
1/4 pt	vegetable stock	150 ml
1/2 oz	soft margarine	15 g
1/2 oz	plain flour	15 g
1/2 pt	skimmed or semi-skimmed milk	275 ml
	salt and freshly ground black pepper	
3 oz	cheddar, grated	75 g
6-8	sheets no-pre-cook lasagne	6-8

Heat the oil in a non-stick saucepan and cook the onions and mushrooms for 5 minutes until soft. Add the baked beans, tomato purée and stock and mix well. Set aside until required.

Melt the margarine, in a saucepan, stir in the flour and cook for 1 minute, stirring. Gradually add the milk and cook over a moderate heat, whisking continuously until the sauce thickens. Season to taste and add half the cheese, stirring well to mix.

Spoon half the baked bean mixture over the base of a 9-inch (23-cm) square ovenproof dish. Cover with half the lasagne. Repeat the layers once more, ending with a layer of lasagne. Spoon over the cheese sauce to cover the lasagne completely. Sprinkle with the remaining cheese and place in a preheated oven at 190°C (375°F) Gas Mark 5 for approximately 25-30 minutes, until golden brown. Serves 4-6.

PER SERVING	
calories	380
g fat	16
g protein	17
g carbohydrate	46

Scrummy Sandwich Fillings

Here are some ideas for quick and easy lunch-box sandwiches that will have the children shouting 'Scrummy Yummy'.

Tuna and Cheese

1	can (7 oz/200 g) tuna in brine or water, drained and flaked	1
1 oz	cheddar, grated	25 g
3 tbsp	salad cream	45 ml

Mix the ingredients together well. This filling is enough to make four rounds of sandwiches, which is 8 slices of bread.

TOTAL FOR 4 ROUNDS (Filling Only)	
calories	418
g fat	20
g protein	51
g carbohydrate	0

Egg and Salad Cream

2	hard-boiled eggs, finely chopped	2
3 tbsp	salad cream	45 ml
	salt and pepper to taste	

Mix the egg and salad cream together and season lightly. This filling will make enough for three rounds of sandwiches, which is 6 slices of bread.

TOTAL FOR 3 ROUNDS (Filling Only)	
calories	342
g fat	28
g protein	15
g carbohydrate	0

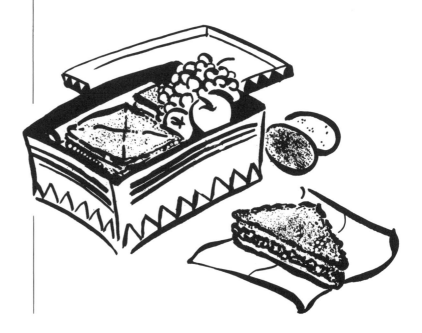

Sail Boats

Children can impress their friends when they come to tea with these sail boats as they are easy and fun to make.

1	can (7 oz/200 g) tuna in brine or water	1
3 tbsp	salad cream	45 ml
6	small bridge rolls	6
2-inch	piece cucumber	5-cm
1/4	red pepper, cut into squares	1/4
1	stick celery	1
12	cocktail sticks	12

Carefully open the can of tuna (or ask an adult to help you) and drain off the liquid. Place the tuna in a mixing bowl and mash with a fork. Add the salad cream and mix together well.

Cut the rolls in half lengthways and spread each half with the tuna mixture. Slice the cucumber lengthways to make rectangles. Cut each slice in half to make a triangle for the sail. Thread the cucumber sails on to cocktail sticks and top each stick with a square of red pepper for a flag.

Stick the sails into the centre of the rolls. Cut the celery stick into small pieces to make the rudder for each boat. Place at the back of each boat. Makes 12 boats.

PER BOAT	
calories	80
g fat	2
g protein	6
g carbohydrate	10

You could also use cutters such as animals or those used for making gingerbread men.

Toasted Houses

Making toast into houses and creating a picture makes a light lunch or snack much more exciting!

4	medium slices bread	4
1 oz	soft margarine	25 g
1 1/2 oz	peanut butter	40 g
3 oz	cheddar cheese	75 g

Toast the bread until golden brown. Cut diagonally across the two top corners of each slice of toast to make a roof shape.

Cut a rectangle out of the bottom of each slice for the door and use this piece to make a chimney. Spread each piece of toast thinly with margarine and peanut butter. Cut the cheese into slices and make three squares for each piece of toast, for the windows. You will need 12 squares of cheese altogether. Serve straight away. Makes 4 houses.

PER HOUSE	
calories	210
g fat	11
g protein	12
g carbohydrate	15

Suitable for freezing.
After adding the sauce and
grated cheese, cool and freeze.
Defrost thoroughly and then
bake at 180°C (350°F) Gas
Mark 4 for 20-25 minutes until
piping hot and golden brown.

Thirty-Minute Macaroni

As a working mother I welcome any dish which you can
prepare in advance, place in the fridge and have little
cooking to do when you come home. If you want to substitute
8 oz/225 g of peas in place of the sweetcorn, this would give a
total of 36 g carbohydrate per serving for 4 people, or 29 g
carbohydrate if serving 5 people.

1 lb	lean minced beef	450 g
1	large onion, chopped	1
2	large carrots, diced	2
1 tbsp	dried mixed herbs	15 ml
2 tbsp	tomato purée	30 ml
1/4 pt	hot beef stock	150 ml
1	can (14 oz/400 g) chopped tomatoes	1
1	can (7 oz/200 g) sweetcorn	1
	salt and freshly ground black pepper	
7 oz	macaroni or pasta shapes	200 g
1 oz	soft margarine	25 g
1 oz	plain flour	25 g
1/2 pt	semi-skimmed milk	275 ml
4 oz	cheddar, grated	100 g

Place the minced beef, onion and carrots in a large non-stick
pan and cook for 5 minutes, stirring occasionally until the meat
has browned. Drain off any excess fat. Return to the heat and
stir in the herbs, purée, stock and tomatoes. Bring to the boil,
cover and simmer for 15 minutes. Add the sweetcorn and cook
for a further 5 minutes. Season to taste.

Meanwhile, boil the pasta in lightly salted boiling water
according to the packet instructions.

Place the margarine, flour and milk in a saucepan and whisk
continuously over a moderate heat until the sauce thickens. Stir
in three quarters of the cheese over a low heat until melted.
Season to taste.

Pour the minced beef mixture into an ovenproof dish. Drain
the pasta and arrange over the mince. Spoon the sauce over the
top to cover. Sprinkle with the remaining cheese. Grill under a
preheated grill for 5-10 minutes or until golden brown and
heated through. Serve hot with salad or freshly cooked
vegetables. Serves 4.

PER SERVING	
calories	659
g fat	24
g protein	50
g carbohydrate	66

Serve with Dry Roasted Potatoes (page 208), Bread Sauce (page 209) and freshly cooked vegetables.

Traditional Roast Chicken with Sultana and Parsley Stuffing

Most children like a traditional Sunday roast dinner. This not only tastes delicious but is surprisingly low in fat too. Use the cooking liquid from the accompanying vegetables in place of the chicken stock if desired. Removing the skin from the chicken when carving will make the meal even lower in fat.

5¼ lb	chicken	2.4 kg
1	large onion	1
1 oz	sultanas	25 g
4 oz	fresh breadcrumbs	100 g
6 tbsp	chopped fresh parsley	90 ml
1¼ pt	water or chicken stock	700 ml
1 tbsp	cornflour	15 ml
	salt and freshly ground black pepper	

Rinse the chicken cavity with cold water and drain well. Finely chop the onion and place in a food processor. Mix in the sultanas, breadcrumbs and parsley and process for a few seconds until the mixture binds together. Season to taste.

Lift up the skin around the neck end of the chicken. Ease the skin away from the flesh and gently push the stuffing underneath. Tuck the neck skin under the chicken and truss the bird loosely with string.

Place the chicken in a roasting tin, cover with foil and cook at 190°C (375°F) Gas Mark 5 for 20 minutes per 1 lb (450 g), plus 20 minutes extra. Remove the foil from the chicken 30 minutes before the end of cooking time.

Test the chicken by inserting a skewer into the thickest part of the leg. If the juices run clear it is ready. Transfer to a serving plate.

Make the gravy: Drain the fat from the roasting tin and discard. Mix the cornflour with 2 tbsp (30 ml) of cold water until smooth. Pour into the roasting tin. Pour the water or chicken stock into the tin and stir occasionally over a low heat until slightly thickened. (This makes a thin gravy.) Serve with the carved chicken. Serves 6.

PER SERVING	
calories	249
g fat	7
g protein	33
g carbohydrate	14

Peach Crunch

A simple dessert which can easily be made up by children themselves, with the help of an adult to purée the peaches. Substitute other tinned fruit such as apricots, pears or mandarins instead of peaches for a variation.

1	can (14 oz/400 g) peach slices in natural juice	1
3 tbsp	granulated artificial sweetener or caster sugar (or to taste)	45 ml
1	carton (1 lb/450 g) virtually-fat-free fromage frais	1
4	Hob Nob or digestive biscuits, roughly crushed	4

Drain the peaches, reserving the juice. Place the peaches and 2 tablespoons of the juice in a liquidiser or food processor and blend to a smooth purée. Stir in 2 tablespoons of sugar or sweetener (or to taste).

Stir the remaining sweetener into the fromage frais. Layer the peach purée and fromage frais in 4-5 glasses. Crumble the biscuits over the top and chill in the refrigerator until required. Serves 4.

PER SERVING	
calories	165
g fat	3
g protein	10
g carbohydrate	26

Peach Melba Shake
Use a large ripe peach and a raspberry yogurt.

Strawberry Milkshake

Make sure that the milk is ice-cold before you make the milkshake so that it can be served while it is frothy. Add a little artificial sweetener if you like to give a sweeter taste.

6 oz	fresh strawberries, hulled	175 g
1	carton (4½ oz/125 g) strawberry yogurt	1
1 pt	semi-skimmed milk	550 ml

Place all the ingredients in a liquidiser and process for a few seconds until smooth and frothy. Pour into tall glasses and serve straight away. Serves 4.

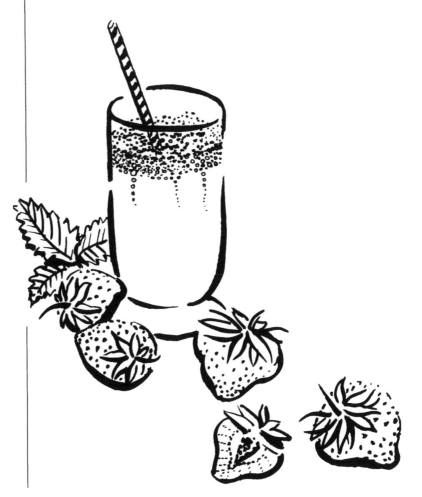

PER SERVING	
calories	107
g fat	3
g protein	7
g carbohydrate	15

Moon Rock Buns

Younger children will enjoy making these buns but may need some help from an adult to cook them, especially when they are handling hot equipment.

8 oz	self-raising white flour	200 g
4 oz	soft margarine	100 g
2 oz	granulated sugar	50 g
2 oz	currants or sultanas	50 g
1	egg, beaten	1
5 tbsp	skimmed milk	75 ml

Ask an adult to turn on the oven to 200°C (400°F) Gas Mark 6. Place the flour in a sieve over a mixing bowl and sieve. Rub the margarine into the flour with your thumb and fingertips until the mixture looks like breadcrumbs. Stir in the sugar and the currants or sultanas.

Place the egg and milk in a small bowl and beat together with a fork. Pour into the currant mixture in the mixing bowl. Mix well with a wooden spoon (the mixture will be sticky).

Lightly brush a baking tray with oil to grease it. This prevents the mixture sticking to the tray during cooking. Place 14 spoonfuls of the mixture spaced apart on the baking tray. Bake the rock buns in the oven for 10-15 minutes. (Now is the time to clear up any mess!) Ask an adult to take the buns out of the oven for you when they are golden brown. If you are allowed to do it yourself, be very careful. Always wear oven gloves when you put your hands in the oven. Place the buns on a cooling rack to cool. Makes 14 buns.

PER BUN	
calories	132
g fat	7
g protein	2
g carbohydrate	17

Tropical Island Biscuits

Have fun making these biscuits and then share them with your family or friends.

4 oz	self-raising flour	100 g
1 oz	caster sugar	25 g
2 oz	desiccated coconut	50 g
1	egg	1
2 oz	soft margarine	50 g

   Ask an adult to turn on the oven at 200°C (400°F) Gas Mark 6. Place the flour, sugar and coconut in a mixing bowl and mix with a wooden spoon. Break the egg into a small bowl and beat with a fork. Melt the margarine gently in a saucepan, or ask an adult to do this for you.

   Gradually add the egg and the margarine to the flour mixture and mix to a firm dough. (You may not need to add all of the liquid.)

   Lightly brush a baking tray with oil to grease it. Shape the biscuit mixture into 10 or 12 round balls and place spaced apart on the baking tray. Bake the biscuits in the oven for 10-15 minutes.

   Ask an adult to take the biscuits out of the oven for you when they are golden brown. If you are allowed to do it yourself, be very careful. Always wear oven gloves when you put your hands in the oven. Place the biscuits on a cooling rack to cool. Makes 10.

PER BISCUIT	
calories	120
g fat	8
g protein	2
g carbohydrate	11

Bread Hedgehogs

It doesn't take very long to make the hedgehog shapes and it will be worth the effort when you present these to your children. They could also help you shape the dough. Why not try different shapes? Teddy bear faces or other animals such as mice are great fun too.

1 lb	strong wholemeal bread flour	450 g
1½ tsp	salt	7.5 ml
1	sachet easy-blend dried yeast	1
½ pt	warmed milk	275 ml
28	currants	28

In a large bowl, mix together the flour, salt and yeast. Pour in the warmed milk and mix to make a firm dough. Knead until smooth and springy. Place the dough in a bowl, cover with a clean tea towel and leave to prove in a warm place for 1-1½ hours or until doubled in size.

Remove the dough from the bowl and knead again for 2 minutes. Cut into 14 pieces and form into oval shapes with a pointed nose. Snip the top of the dough with scissors to make spikes. Press two currants into the dough to make eyes. Cover again and leave in a warm place for 20-30 minutes until doubled in size. Brush with a little milk and bake in a preheated oven at 220°C (425°F) Gas Mark 7 for 10-15 minutes or until risen and golden brown. Serve warm. Makes 14.

PER HEDGEHOG	
calories	109
g fat	1
g protein	5
g carbohydrate	22

Birthday Party Menu for small children

Sail Boats (page 191) Crispy Scotch Eggs (page 186) or Scrummy Sandwiches (page 190)
Cucumber, carrot and celery sticks, cherry tomatoes and raisins
Dreamy Fruit Jelly (page 203) or Raspberry Ice (page 176)
Birthday Cake (page 199)

Party Menu for older children

Quick Tomato Salsa (page 26) with tortilla chips
Spicy Chicken Satay with Creamy Peanut Dip (page 29)
Herb and Garlic Bread (page 30)
Courgette, Sweetcorn and Red Pepper Pizza (page 71), served with a selection of salads
Summer Fruit Layers (page 166)
Birthday Cake (page 199 or 215)

Birthday Cakes

Most children love to have a special cake for their birthday and this is often the centrepiece of the tea table. The cake is usually a basic sponge or fruit cake and it can be decorated in many different ways. Why not try the Victoria Sandwich Cake (page 200)?

Marzipan or fondant icing may be used to cover the cake as well as moulded into various decorative shapes. It can easily be coloured by kneading in edible food colourings to give a bright appearance or bought ready coloured.

It is unlikely that a large slice of Birthday cake will be eaten during the party as it is often cut up and taken home in a party bag. You could encourage your child to eat his or her slice of cake at the end of a meal or include it as part of a snack the following day. In this way your child can still enjoy a special day without too much effect on his or her blood glucose level.

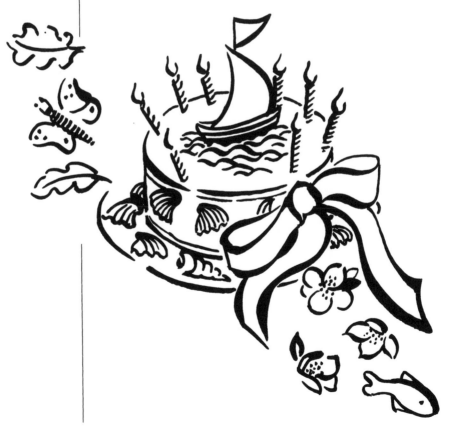

Store in an airtight container.
Best eaten within 2-3 days.
Suitable for freezing.

Victoria Sandwich Cake

This is one of the first cakes that I learnt to make when I was a young girl. It is a versatile mixture which can be used as the basis for so many recipes, from elaborate Birthday cakes to simple cup cakes or sponge puddings. You can add many different flavours such as cocoa powder, lemon or orange rind or coffee.

6 oz	soft margarine	175 g
3 oz	caster sugar	75 g
3	eggs, lightly beaten	3
6 oz	self-raising flour	175 g
1/2 tsp	baking powder	2.5 ml
	a few drops vanilla essence	
2 tbsp	hot water	30 ml

Cream the margarine and sugar together until pale and creamy. Add the eggs, a little at a time, beating well after each addition. Sift the flour and baking powder. Using a metal spoon, lightly fold in half the flour mixture, then carefully fold in the remainder with the vanilla essence and water.

Divide the mixture between two lightly greased and base-lined 7-inch (18-cm) sandwich tins. Bake at 190°C (375°F) Gas Mark 5 in the centre of the oven for approximately 20-25 minutes or until golden and firm to the touch. Turn out and cool on a wire rack. Serves 8-10.

Fill the cake with jam or fruit and cream/fromage frais.

PER SERVING	
calories	223/178
g fat	11/9
g protein	6/5
g carbohydrate	25/20

Festive

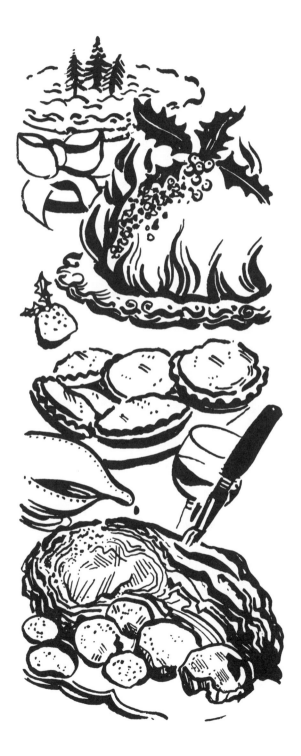

Christmas is a time for enjoyment, there is no need for special recipes or foods. Everyone over-indulges at Christmas and the occasional high BG reading will not upset your long-term control. With a little care and forward planning you can enjoy the festive season and stay in control of your diabetes. This chapter includes recipes for most of the traditional Christmas foods including a delicious Christmas cake. The recipes can all be enjoyed by the whole family.

Cranberry Sauce

Fresh cranberries are usually available in supermarkets just before Christmas.

9 oz	fresh cranberries, topped and tailed	250 g
1	orange, grated rind and juice	1
5 tbsp	water	90 ml
2-3 tbsp	sugar to taste	30-45 ml

Place the cranberries, orange rind and juice and water in a saucepan. Simmer for 15 minutes, or until the berries are tender. Remove from the heat and add the sugar to taste. Serves 6-8.

PER SERVING	
calories	17/12
g fat	0
g protein	0
g carbohydrate	neg

Roast Pheasant

Many people like to serve pheasant at Christmas instead of turkey, particularly if there are not too many to cater for. This recipe uses a brace (pair) of oven-ready pheasants which will serve 4 people.

2	oven-ready pheasants	2
2 oz	lean back bacon, rind removed	50 g
1/2 oz	soft margarine	15 g
1 tbsp	plain flour	15 ml
1/2 pt	boiling chicken stock	275 ml
	salt and freshly ground black pepper	

Truss the birds and cover the breasts with bacon. Place a knob of the margarine inside each bird. Place the birds side by side in a large roasting tin. Roast in a preheated oven at 200°C (400°F) Gas Mark 6 for 50 minutes. Baste frequently with the cooking sauces during cooking. 5 minutes before the end of cooking time, remove the bacon and discard.

Place the pheasants on a heated serving dish and remove the trussing strings. Keep hot. Meanwhile, skim the fat from the cooking juices. Stir in the flour and gradually add the stock. Boil on the hob for 2-3 minutes and season to taste. Serve the gravy with the pheasants. Serve with boiled new potatoes and freshly cooked seasonal vegetables. Serves 4.

If you are put off pheasant because of plucking the feathers, my brother-in-law, Mark, gave me this tip. Pluck a few feathers from the breast of the bird and slit the skin. The skin can then be pulled off complete with the feathers, which saves a lot of work.

PER SERVING	
calories	329
g fat	16
g protein	43
g carbohydrate	4

Peppered Roast Beef

Roast beef is ideal to serve on Boxing Day or to have as extra meat with turkey. This hot spicy coating gives the beef a rich flavour and not adding extra oil during cooking makes a healthier meal.

3½ lb	lean topside of beef	1.5 kg
3 tbsp	crushed mixed peppercorns	45 ml
6 tbsp	horseradish sauce	90 ml
2 tbsp	gravy powder	30 ml
2 tbsp	cold water	30 ml
	salt and freshly ground black pepper	

Trim the beef of any excess fat, and wipe the joint with kitchen paper. Mix the peppercorns and horseradish sauce together to form a paste. Spread the paste over the meat and place on a trivet set in a roasting pan. Cover with foil and cook at 220°C (425°F) Gas Mark 7 for 15 minutes per lb (450 g), plus 15 min, for rare, 20 min per 1 lb (450 g), plus 20 min for medium, and 25 min per 1 lb (450 g), plus 25 min for well done.

Remove the joint from the oven and stand covered on a warmed serving plate for about 10 minutes before carving.

Drain away the excess fat from the roasting tin. Mix the gravy powder with the cold water to form a smooth paste. Stir the paste into the pan juices with 1 pt (550 ml) of cooking liquid strained from accompanying vegetables. Simmer on the hob, stirring continuously until the gravy is thickened. Season to taste.

Serve the roast beef with potatoes and freshly cooked vegetables. Serves 8.

PER SERVING	
calories	310
g fat	9
g protein	55
g carbohydrate	2

Normandy Apple Flan

Even though I have adapted this dessert from the traditional recipe to lower the fat and calories, it is still rather high for an everyday meal. However, it does make a nice dessert when entertaining, or as an occasional treat. It is best served warm.

6 oz	plain flour	175 g
	a pinch of salt	
6 oz	soft margarine	175 g
2 tbsp	sugar	30 ml
2	eggs	2
½ oz	cornflour	15 g
4 oz	ground almonds	100 g
¼ tsp	almond essence	1.25 ml
1½ lb	cooking apples	550 g
2 tbsp	apricot jam	30 ml
2 tbsp	water	30 ml

Sift the flour and salt into a bowl. Rub in half the margarine until the mixture resembles fine breadcrumbs. Add enough cold water to mix to a soft dough. Wrap in greaseproof paper and chill for 30 minutes.

Meanwhile, beat the remaining fat with the sugar. Beat in the eggs, cornflour, ground almonds and essence. Roll out the pastry on a lightly floured board to line a 9-inch (23-cm) fluted flan tin. Prick the base and bake blind at 200°C (400°F) Gas Mark 6 for 10 minutes. Remove the baking beans and paper, and cook for a further 5 minutes. Set aside to cool.

Spread the almond cream over the cooled pastry base. Peel, core and thinly slice the apples. Arrange over the cream. Cook at 200°C (400°F) Gas Mark 6 for 8 minutes. Reduce the heat to 180°C (350°F) Gas Mark 4 and cook for a further 15-20 minutes until golden.

Melt the apricot jam and water together in a small saucepan. Remove the tart from the tin and brush with the apricot glaze. Serve warm with a little half-fat cream or fromage frais. Serves 10.

PER SERVING	
calories	285
g fat	21
g protein	5
g carbohydrate	20

Pineapple
Some varieties of pineapple have a green skin but are still perfectly ripe. A pineapple is ripe if a leaf can be pulled from the crown with one sharp tug.

PER SERVING	
calories	80
g fat	0
g protein	2
g carbohydrate	20

Tropical Paradise Fruit Salad

Exotic fruits such as mango and lychee are now readily available from supermarkets or local markets. This is a refreshing dessert which has no fat and is low in calories.

2	small oranges, peeled and segmented	2
2	kiwi fruit, peeled and sliced	2
1	small pineapple, skin removed and diced	1
1	small ripe mango, peeled, stone removed and diced	1
1	galia melon, peeled and diced	1
4	lychees, skin and stone removed, halved	4
4 fl oz	unsweetened orange juice	100 ml
4 fl oz	diet lemonade	100 ml
2 tbsp	rum (optional)	30 ml

Place all the fruit in a large bowl and toss lightly to mix. Pour over the orange juice, lemonade and rum if using. Cover and chill for 1-2 hours. Serve chilled. Serves 6.

Raspberry Trifle

A mixture of summer fruits may be used in place of the raspberries. For a burst of summer in the middle of winter, I use a frozen packet which includes raspberries, redcurrants, blackcurrants and strawberries.

8 oz	raspberries, defrosted and drained if frozen	225 g
1	sachet raspberry flavour sugar-free jelly crystals	1
2 tbsp	custard powder	30 ml
1/2 pt	skimmed milk	275 ml
2 tbsp	granulated artificial sweetener or caster sugar	30 ml
1	carton (5 fl oz/142 ml) whipping cream, whipped	1
1/2 oz	toasted flaked almonds	15 g

PER SERVING	
calories	152
g fat	11
g protein	3
g carbohydrate	10

Place the fruit in the base of a serving bowl. Make up the jelly crystals according to the directions on the packet and make up to 1 pint (550 ml) with cold water. Pour the jelly on to the fruit and place in the refrigerator to set. Make up the custard using the custard powder and milk. Remove from the heat and sweeten with sugar or artificial sweetener to taste. Allow to cool before pouring over the set jelly. Spread the whipped cream over the custard and chill. Sprinkle with the toasted nuts just before serving. Serves 6-8.

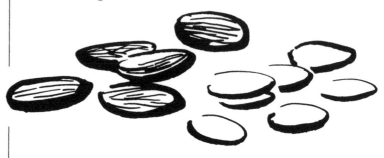

Serve with Custard (page 172) or half-fat cream.

Christmas Pudding

A moist pudding with no added sugar which still tastes rich and delicious as the sweetness comes from the fruit.

4 oz	plain wholemeal flour	100 g
¼ tsp	salt	1.25 ml
½ tsp	ground nutmeg	2.5 ml
½ tsp	ground mixed spice	2.5 ml
4 oz	soft margarine	100 g
2	eggs, beaten	2
1	lemon, grated rind and juice	1
2 tbsp	brandy	30 ml
1	small eating apple, cored and finely grated	1
2	large carrots, finely grated	2
4 oz	wholemeal breadcrumbs	100 g
2 oz	chopped mixed nuts	50 g
2 oz	glacé cherries, rinsed, dried and chopped	50 g
6 oz	currants	175 g
6 oz	sultanas	175 g
8 oz	raisins	225 g

In a large bowl, sift together the flour, salt and spices, tipping any bran remaining in the sieve back into the bowl. Stir in all the remaining ingredients and mix well until thoroughly combined. Spoon into two 1½-pint (825-ml) lightly greased pudding basins. Cover with a double thickness of buttered greaseproof paper with a pleat in, then with a layer of pleated foil. Secure with string. Steam the puddings in a large steamer over a pan of gently simmering water for 4½ hours. Leave to cool, then cover with fresh greaseproof paper and foil. Store in a cool, dry place for up to two weeks. To reheat, steam for 1½-2 hours. Makes two 1½-pint (825-ml) puddings. Each pudding serves 10.

PER SERVING	
calories	160
g fat	7
g protein	2
g carbohydrate	23

Dreamy Fruit Jelly

This is an easy dessert to make yet looks impressive if set in a decorative jelly mould and decorated with fresh summer fruits. I like to serve this with strawberries, raspberries, redcurrants and blackcurrants, grown in my mother's garden and full of flavour.

½ pt	boiling water	275 ml
1	sachet sugar-free raspberry jelly	1
1	sachet sugar-free Dream Topping	1
¼ pt	skimmed milk	150 ml
5 fl oz	carton raspberry yogurt	150 g
8 oz	frozen mixed summer fruits or raspberries	225 g

Pour the boiling water into a measuring jug, add the jelly and stir to dissolve. Set aside to cool slightly.

Meanwhile, in a large bowl, make up the Dream Topping with the milk according to the packet instructions. Fold in the yogurt. Separate the summer fruit or raspberries – there is no need to thaw the fruit completely – and stir into the jelly. Stir the jelly into the dream topping mixture and mix thoroughly.

Pour the mixture into a serving bowl. Place in the refrigerator for a few hours to set. Serves 6.

PER SERVING	
calories	62
g fat	3
g protein	2
g carbohydrate	8

Herby Yorkshires
Add ½ teaspoon dried mixed herbs to the batter.

Mini Yorkshire Puddings

4 oz	plain flour	100 g
1	egg, beaten	1
½ pt	skimmed milk	275 ml
4 tbsp	olive or sunflower oil	60 ml
	salt and freshly ground black pepper	

Sift the flour into a bowl. Beat the egg and milk together. Make a well in the centre of the flour and beat in the egg and milk until smooth. Allow the mixture to stand for 15 minutes.

Heat the oil in a 12-section bun tin in the oven for a few minutes. Quickly pour the batter evenly into the bun tray. Cook at 220°C (425°F) Gas Mark 7 for 20-25 minutes until risen and golden. Makes 12.

PER SERVING	
calories	82
g fat	5
g protein	2
g carbohydrate	7

Dry Roasted Potatoes

Roast potatoes without the fat! These potatoes are a mini version of baked potatoes with a crunchy outside and soft potato in the centre. They are best served with a roast dinner with gravy, otherwise they may seem rather dry.

2½ lb	potatoes, peeled and halved	1.1 kg
2 tsp	ground paprika	10 ml

Parboil the potatoes in lightly salted boiling water for 10 minutes. Drain well and turn into a roasting tin. Sprinkle the paprika over the potatoes and mix well to coat. Cook in the bottom of the oven at 220°C (425°F) Gas Mark 7 for 1 hour 10 minutes, turning several times during cooking. Serves 6.

PER SERVING	
calories	138
g fat	0
g protein	4
g carbohydrate	31

Bread Sauce

Bread sauce just isn't the same with wholemeal bread so I use white breadcrumbs. As it is served as an accompaniment to a roast dinner, the amount of fibre it would contribute would be minimal anyway.

1	medium onion, peeled and halved	1
3	cloves	3
1 pt	milk	550 ml
1	bay leaf	1
4 oz	fresh white breadcrumbs	100 g
	salt and freshly ground black pepper	
1/2 oz	butter	15 g
	a pinch of grated nutmeg	

Stud the onion with cloves and place in a saucepan with the milk and bay leaf. Bring to the boil, then immediately remove from the heat. Allow to stand for 30 minutes.

Discard the onion and bay leaf. Stir in the breadcrumbs and season well with salt and black pepper. Cook over a gentle heat for 5-10 minutes, stirring continuously until the bread sauce has thickened. Remove from the heat and stir in the butter. Pour into a serving jug, sprinkle with a little nutmeg and serve. Serves 8.

PER SERVING	
calories	94
g fat	5
g protein	4
g carbohydrate	10

Suitable for freezing. Cool and pack into a rigid container to freeze. Defrost and then warm in a hot oven for 3-4 minutes before serving.

Mince Pies

Use a star cutter to decorate the mince pies or alternatively you could use a holly cutter if you have one. I always make my pastry in a food processor which gives a shorter texture and makes handling easier.

For the pastry

6 oz	plain flour	150 g
3 oz	soft margarine	75 g
	cold water to bind	

For the filling

12-16 tsp	mincemeat	60-80 ml
	a little milk for glazing	
	a little sugar (optional)	

Make the pastry and allow to chill in a refrigerator for 30 minutes. Roll out on a lightly floured board. Using 2½-inch (6-cm) cutter and a small star cutter, cut out an equal number of bases and stars.

Place the pastry circles in patty tins and put 1 teaspoon (5 ml) of mincemeat into each. Place a star top on each pie. Bake in a preheated oven at 200°C (400°F) Gas Mark 6 for 10-15 minutes. Brush with a little milk and sprinkle with a little sugar if desired when the pies come out of the oven. Serve warm. Makes 12.

PER MINCE PIE	
calories	107
g fat	5
g protein	1
g carbohydrate	14

Sangria

This will remind you of hot sunny holidays!

1	bottle (75 cl) dry red wine	1
3/4 pt	unsweetened orange juice	425 ml
1	bottle (2 pt/1 litre) low-calorie lemonade	1
	a few orange slices	
	ice cubes	

Mix the ingredients together in a large jug or punch bowl. Add the orange slices and ice. Serve chilled. Serves 10.

PER SERVING	
calories	67
g fat	0
g protein	0
g carbohydrate	4

Apricot Choux Ring

An alternative dessert for those who dislike Christmas pudding. The choux pastry ring may be made and baked ahead of time and frozen. Ring the changes by using canned peaches, mandarins or fresh fruit for the filling in place of apricots.

For the pastry		
1/4 pt	water	150 ml
2 oz	soft margarine	50 g
2 1/2 oz	plain flour, sieved	65 g
2	eggs beaten	2
For the filling		
7 oz	reduced-fat soft cheese	200 g
1	carton (5 oz/150 g) yogurt, peach or orange flavour	1
1	can (14 oz/400 g) apricot halves in natural juice, drained and roughly chopped	1
	a little sugar to serve	

To freeze: Wrap the unfilled choux ring well after cooling and freeze for up to three months.

Place the water and margarine in a saucepan and heat gently until it melts. Bring to a rapid boil then remove from the heat. Add the flour all at once and beat hard with a wooden spoon until the mixture leaves the sides of the pan clean. Gradually add the beaten eggs until the mixture is smooth and glossy, leaving a little left for brushing. Pipe or spoon the mixture on to a lightly greased baking sheet to form a 7-inch (18-cm) circle. Brush all over with the remaining beaten egg. Bake in a preheated oven at 220°C (425°F) Gas Mark 7 for 10 minutes. Then reduce the heat and cook at 200°C (400°F) Gas Mark 6 for a further 15-20 minutes. Remove from the oven and slit in half, horizontally.

Return both halves to the oven, opened side up for a further 3-4 minutes to dry out the centre. Cool on a cooling rack.

Beat together the soft cheese and yogurt for the filling. Add the chopped apricot and mix well. Use to fill the base of the choux ring, then top with the lid. Sprinkle with a little sugar to serve. Serves 6-8.

PER SERVING	
calories	190/143
g fat	11/8
g protein	8/6
g carbohydrate	16/12

Glacé Fruit Bombe

This dessert makes a delicious and refreshing alternative to Christmas pudding.

1	sachet (0.4 oz/11 g) gelatine	1
2 tbsp	water	30 ml
1	can (6 oz/170 g) evaporated milk, chilled overnight	1
8 oz	low-fat fromage frais	225 g
1 tbsp	sugar	15 ml
4 oz	seedless raisins	100 g
2 tbsp	brandy	30 ml
2 oz	glacé cherries, washed and halved	50 g

Dissolve the gelatine in the water in a bowl set over a pan of gently simmering water. Set aside to cool. Whisk the evaporated milk in a chilled bowl until double in size and stiff peaks form. Fold the cooled gelatine into the evaporated milk together with the fromage frais and sugar. Place in a shallow tray and freeze for 1 hour or until partially set. Soak the raisins in the brandy.

Turn milk mixture into a bowl and whisk thoroughly. Beat in the glacé cherries and soaked raisins. Place in a lightly greased 2-pint (1-litre) pudding basin. Freeze overnight or until solid. Remove from the freezer 5 minutes before serving. Turn out on to a serving plate and serve immediately. Serves 6.

PER SERVING	
calories	144
g fat	3
g protein	7
g carbohydrate	22

Mini Christmas Puddings

Even a reduced-sugar Christmas pudding is still rather high in calories and carbohydrate. However, a serving on Christmas day is perfectly acceptable. It is the long term control which is important.

4 oz	ready-to-eat dried apricots, finely chopped	100 g
4 oz	sultanas, washed	100 g
4 oz	seedless raisins, washed	100 g
4 tbsp	brandy	60 ml
1 oz	glacé cherries, washed and quartered	25 g
2 oz	chopped mixed nuts	50 g
3 oz	fresh breadcrumbs	75 g
2 oz	suet or vegetarian suet	50 g
1 tsp	ground mixed spice	5 ml
½ tsp	ground cinnamon	2.5 ml
1	lemon, grated rind	1
2	eggs, lightly beaten	2

Grease and base-line 8 dariole moulds or very small, heatproof teacups.

Soak the dried apricots, sultanas and raisins in the brandy overnight. Add the cherries and nuts. Mix together the breadcrumbs, suet, spices and lemon rind, then stir into the fruit mixture. Finally, add the eggs and stir well to mix thoroughly. Divide the mixture among the prepared moulds. Cover each with greaseproof paper and foil, then tie securely with string.

Steam the puddings in a large steamer over a pan of gently simmering water for 2 hours. Leave to cool, then cover with fresh greaseproof paper and foil. Store for up to two weeks.

To reheat, steam for a further 2 hours. Makes 8 puddings.

PER SERVING	
calories	239
g fat	10
g protein	5
g carbohydrate	30

Wrap in greaseproof paper and foil and store in an airtight container. Best eaten within 2 weeks. Suitable for freezing.

Halfway through the storage the cake may be unwrapped and the base pricked several times with a skewer. Drizzle 2 tablespoons of brandy over the base. Re-wrap.

This cake may be decorated for special occasions in the traditional way using marzipan and fondant or royal icing (remember to add the extra carbohydrate to the total for the cake). For birthdays, anniversaries etc. there is no reason why a person with diabetes should not enjoy a small piece of cake along with everyone else. This may be eaten at the end of a high-fibre meal or included as a snack.

PER SERVING	
calories	133
g fat	6
g protein	2
g carbohydrate	20

Celebration Cake

At Diabetes UK, we have many calls or letters asking for a fruit cake recipe. This special occasion cake is great for Christmas.

5 oz	plain flour	150 g
1/2 tsp	salt	2.5 ml
1 tsp	cinnamon	5 ml
1 tsp	mixed spice	5 ml
1/2 tsp	grated nutmeg	2.5 ml
8 oz	raisins	225 g
8 oz	currants	225 g
8 oz	sultanas	225 g
4 oz	glacé cherries, rinsed, dried and quartered	100 g
4 oz	flaked almonds	100 g
5 oz	soft margarine	150 g
2 oz	soft brown sugar	50 g
4	eggs, beaten	4
3 tbsp	brandy	45 ml
1 tsp	bicarbonate of soda	5 ml
2 tsp	warm water	10 ml
2 tbsp	additional brandy (optional)	30 ml

Grease and line an 8-inch (20-cm) round or 7-inch (18-cm) square cake tin with a double thickness of greaseproof paper. Tie a double thickness of newspaper around the outside.

Sift together the flour, salt and spices. Mix together the fruit and nuts. Cream the margarine and sugar together until pale and creamy. Gradually beat in the eggs, adding a tablespoon of flour with each egg. Fold in the remaining flour, fruit and brandy. Mix the bicarbonate of soda with the warm water and add to the mixture. Spoon the mixture into the prepared tin and level the surface. Make a slight dip in the centre with the back of a spoon. Place in a preheated oven at 150°C (300°F) Gas Mark 2 for approximately 2½ hours or until a skewer inserted comes out clean. Cover the cake with foil or several thicknesses of brown paper if it starts to become too brown. Cool in the tin for 30 minutes. Turn out on to a wire rack, remove the paper and allow to cool completely. Serves 32.

Use to make Mince Pies (page 210).

Make-At-Home Mincemeat

Making your own mincemeat means that you can cut down on the sugar content considerably. This recipe just has the natural sweetness from the dried fruit and fruit juice, which still affects blood glucose levels. However, it will need to be used within two weeks or alternatively it may be frozen in a plastic container.

8 oz	raisins	225 g
8 oz	sultanas	225 g
4 oz	ready-to-eat dried apricots, finely chopped	100 g
4 oz	glacé cherries, rinsed, dried and finely chopped	100 g
2 oz	chopped mixed nuts	50 g
1	large carrot, peeled and finely grated	1
2 oz	shredded suet	50 g
1	lemon, finely grated rind and juice	1
4 tbsp	unsweetened orange juice	60 ml
1 tbsp	brandy or rum (optional)	15 ml

Place all the ingredients together in a large bowl and mix well. Cover and leave for 2 days in the refrigerator, stirring occasionally.

Pack into clean and sterilised jars or a plastic container, cover and store in the refrigerator. Use within two weeks or freeze until required. Makes approximately 2 lb (900 g).

PER 1 lb (450 g)	
calories	1210
g fat	36
g protein	14
g carbohydrate	217

Index